Ultimate Facercise

Ultimate Facercise

The Complete and Balanced
Muscle-Toning Program for Renewed Vitality
and a More Youthful Appearance

Carole Maggio

A Perigee Book

A PERIGEE BOOK
Published by the Penguin Group
Penguin Group (USA) Inc.
375 Hudson Street, New York, New York 10014, USA
Penguin Group (Canada), 90 Eglinton Avenue East, Suite 700,
Toronto, Ontario M4P 2Y3, Canada (a division of Pearson Penguin
Canada Inc.) • Penguin Books Ltd., 80 Strand, London WC2R 0RL,
England • Penguin Group Ireland, 25 St. Stephen's Green, Dublin 2,
Ireland (a division of Penguin Books Ltd.) • Penguin Group (Australia),
250 Camberwell Road, Camberwell, Victoria 3124, Australia
(a division of Pearson Australia Group Pty. Ltd.) • Penguin Books
India Pvt. Ltd., 11 Community Centre, Panchsheel Park,
New Delhi—110 017, India • Penguin Group (NZ), 67 Apollo Drive,
Rosedale, Auckland 0632, New Zealand (a division of Pearson
New Zealand Ltd.) • Penguin Books (South Africa) (Pty.) Ltd.,
24 Sturdee Avenue, Rosebank, Johannesburg 2196, South Africa
Penguin Books Ltd., Registered Offices: 80 Strand,
London WC2R 0RL, England

While the author has made every effort to provide accurate
telephone numbers and Internet addresses at the time of
publication, neither the publisher nor the author assumes any
responsibility for errors or for changes that occur after publication.
Further, the publisher does not have any control over and does not
assume any responsibility for author or third-party websites or their
content.

ULTIMATE FACERCISE

First American edition: July 2011
Originally published as *The Ultimate Facercise* in Great Britain in
2011 by Pan Macmillan.

ISBN: 978-0-399-53667-0
PRINTED IN THE UNITED STATES OF AMERICA

10   9   8   7

Most Perigee books are available at special quantity discounts for
bulk purchases for sales promotions, premiums, fund-raising, or
educational use. Special books, or book excerpts, can also be
created to fit specific needs. For details, write: Special Markets,
Penguin Group (USA) Inc., 375 Hudson Street, New York,
New York 10014.

Publisher's Note

Neither the publisher nor the author is engaged
in rendering professional advice or services to
the individual reader. The ideas, procedures,
and suggestions contained in this book are
not intended as a substitute for consulting
with your physician. All matters regarding your
health require medical supervision. Neither
the author nor the publisher shall be liable or
responsible for any loss or damage allegedly
arising from any information or suggestion in
this book.

Photo Acknowledgments

All exercise photographs by Jenn Kennedy.
P.8 © Plainpicture. P.26 © Yuri Arcurs/
Shutterstock. P.30–32 by Jenn Kennedy. P.38 ©
Efired/Shutterstock. P.50 © Carole Maggio.
P.58 © FotoVeto/Shutterstock. P.84 Efired/
Shutterstock. P.90 © dundanim/Shutterstock. P.98
© Madlen/Shutterstock. P.127 © Ed Ouellette.

Contents

One of my mantras has always been, "You can't help getting older, but you don't have to look older." I know that life is not a dress rehearsal, so why not put your best face forward all the time?

Introduction

If we are truly honest with ourselves, we all want to look and feel our personal best, each and every day of our lives. For some of us, that means exercising our bodies to keep ourselves toned and physically strong. Exercising the body also offers positive mental benefits by making us feel more secure, energetic and optimistic about our lives. But exercising the body will not change our face. Many people look in the mirror and see an image that does not truly reflect how they feel inside. In an attempt to change what they see, they often take drastic measures, such as surgery, only to be disappointed. I am here to tell you that you don't need surgery or chemicals to look as young as you feel – and that you can control what happens to your face as you age. With a little time, dedication and discipline, you too can have a face to match the way you feel inside.

For as long as I can remember, I have had a fascination with beauty. When I was in college, I used to enjoy applying treatments to and makeup on my friends in the dorm, to enhance their natural beauty. We are all given a unique palette to work with and, to me, natural beauty is a radiance and glow that shines from within. It's easy to lose this as we age – as our complexion dulls, our eyes become hooded rather than open, our mouths droop down. But with a little time and dedication, we can restore our own natural beauty. In fact, we can remain beautiful and youthful throughout our entire lives. For me, remaining youthful isn't about looking a certain age, it's about looking the best I can for the age that I am.

Through this book, I hope to offer you the promise of renewed natural beauty by using my Ultimate Facercise program. You don't need to resort to plastic surgery, Botox, fillers and the like to create a more youthful countenance. You do, however, need to set goals for yourself, commit to the plan, perform the exercises correctly and, above all, be consistent and patient.

I'll also advise you on how quality nutrition, proper hydration, healthy lifestyle choices, sun safety and a positive attitude will help keep your skin looking youthful and boost the effect of Facercising. I promise that you will see results if you stick with the program. All you need is 16 minutes a day. So what are you waiting for?

1

What
Facercise
Can Do for You

Before I describe how Facercise can benefit you, and why I believe it is a better option than cosmetic surgery, I want to explain how I created this exercise program – and why I'm living proof that it works!

When I was younger I opted to have plastic surgery on my nose. Unfortunately, the procedure did not turn out as expected, and I was very unhappy with the results. The surgeon left a dent on the side of my nose and the tip was too long. I could have opted to have it redone, but I had lost confidence in his ability to correct it. At the young age of 36, my husband at the time commented that I was "aging beyond my years." Although I knew deep down inside that he was right, I was hurt by his comments and desperately wanted to do something about it. At the time, I was a licensed aesthetician (skincare specialist) and owned a skincare clinic. I offered my clients various treatments, including a massage technique to tone and lift the face. The technique was very popular and worked quite well, but the results were not very long lasting. This got me thinking: "What if I could develop a technique to permanently lift the muscles of the face?" I began experimenting on my own face and developed a program to work the various muscles of the face. The results were positively amazing. Even my coworkers and friends began to take notice. The Facercise program was born.

Throughout the years I have revised, changed and improved upon my program to create even more positive changes in the face. Working the facial muscles against a resistance works in the same manner as lifting weights. You can open up the entire eye area, lift the eyebrows, define and lift the cheeks, plump up your lips, turn mouth corners up, and firm your entire neck and jawline. There is even an exercise to shorten and narrow your nose – or straighten a crooked nose. All you need to do is decide to take control, be disciplined, remain focused and concentrate on the facial muscles while you work them. But, above all, *believe* you *can* and you *will* restore your own natural beauty and youthfulness using my program.

The New Ultimate Facercise Program Is Born

Being the perfectionist that I am, I'm constantly tweaking and improving my program. The original Facercise program (Beginning Facercise) contains 14 synergistic exercises that take only 11 minutes of your time, twice a day, for a total of 22 minutes. Next, I created the Advanced program, which is included in a chapter of *The New Facercise,* which was released in 2002. The Advanced program contains nine exercises to address specific areas of the face that need additional attention, or to create more definition. That program was not meant to replace the Beginning Facercise program, but rather to complement it. The intent was for the Beginning Facercise program to remain the foundation program, from which you can then move on. Since that time, some of my clients have expressed an interest in special exercises, which I've included in the Ultimate Facercise program; for example, the new Nose Transformer exercise (see page 68) to fix a crooked nose, or a nose that curves to one side. Some of my clients have also mentioned their desire for a shortened version of the program. So, some exercises in the new Ultimate Facercise program are replacing older versions and will address more than one area of the face, making this program quicker and more efficient.

Facial-exercise clients of mine, who have trained with me in person or who have trained with me via Skype, know that my program has changed and evolved over the years. Unfortunately, I could not reach out to the millions of people who I have personally trained – or who have read my previous books – to inform them of these improvements. Hence, I decided, after eight years, that it was time for me to write a new book to spread the word. *Ultimate Facercise* is more of a complete and balanced program, utilizing aspects from both the Beginning and Advanced programs. I have tailored this new program using the most advanced face technology, targeting the muscles differently, working them harder and more effectively. Ultimate Facercise, with its 13 synergistic exercises, has replaced the Beginning and Advanced programs, and is now my foundation program. You can start here, without any experience of my previous programs.

Ultimate Facercise is *extreme* Facercise. By this, I mean that your results will be much more dramatic than if you were using my original version of the program. The reason for this is simple. Remember how big and cumbersome mobile phones were in the beginning? They were so large that they almost needed their own zip code – and you practically needed a trolley to haul them around. However, as technology advanced, those large boxes became small smartphones that fit very comfortably in your handbag or pocket. Technology creates better products, and Facercise has kept pace with new technology.

I am now incorporating techniques that utilize the body differently, to create more resistance. More resistance equals faster and better results. In my first book, I explained the importance of the mind–muscle connection. This is still a very important component of my program. In *Ultimate Facercise*, I explain visualization and what that means to your overall success. There are new exercises and subtle changes to old favorites that make a huge difference to the results you will achieve.

When I first wrote *Facercise* and *The New Facercise*, people weren't ready for the detailed instructions necessary to get the most out of my program. Since writing those books, my client base has expanded dramatically. Worldwide, millions of women (and now men, too) are Facercising to keep their faces looking youthful and to address specific issues. Some of the letters, emails and photos I've received from clients have shown remarkable results. I've even received rave reviews from clients who were so inspired and thrilled with their results because it meant that they no longer had to go through the "deeply emotional and financial experience" of surgery that they had been considering. One of those clients is Sharon Martin, who was toying with the idea of the Lifestyle Lift when she found my program. She managed to create some truly wonderful results using my book alone. Now that's quite a testimony!

My clients are from all walks of life, extending around the globe. In fact, Facercise can work for anyone willing to invest just 16 minutes a day. With Ultimate Facercise, you can expect to see results quickly and, as with the foundation program, you will continue to improve upon those results over the weeks, months and even years that you use my program. Remember that old joke about how the second and third days of a new diet are so much easier than the first day, because by this point, you've quit the diet? Don't let Facercise be that kind of thing. Stick to it, and your face (and you) will be glad you did.

Taking the Natural Path

Hardly a day goes by when I don't receive some sort of compliment about my skin – or how remarkable I look for my age. While compliments are always very flattering, the road to natural antiaging isn't easy. Now in my middle-earlies (mid-sixties), I am so very grateful that I've followed the natural path that has allowed me to look as good as I feel.

Many people share my ambition to remain as youthful and vibrant as I can, for as long as I can, but they don't always take the natural path. Perhaps it's my internal instincts that have kept me on the natural path, but it's more likely the result of what I've witnessed over the years in the skincare business. Many of my spa clients have had plastic surgery, Botox, fillers or all of the above before they end up coming to me in distress, panic and dismay. I cannot say that I am totally against plastic surgery. After all, I did have rhinoplasty surgery (albeit a bad one, in my opinion) well before I created the Facercise program. However, all of these procedures come with their own unique, inherent risks. They also come with hefty price tags and need to be repeated (more hefty price tags) over and over again.

I've had clients who have gone under the knife for various procedures and were not at all satisfied with their results. Some felt that although the facelift addressed sagging, they now looked pulled, tight and unnatural. Unfortunately, that's when many feel they need to "hop on the carousel," as I like to say. They elect to get fillers to make their faces appear more full and youthful because, while the facelift addresses the sag, it can't address the loss of fat and collagen under the skin. Fillers will temporarily fill out a hardened-looking face. However, for some, that's an awful lot of filler. Furthermore, it doesn't last very long and needs to be redone on a perpetual basis (the carousel). I have taught clients seeking my help how to build muscles in their faces to actually replace or make up for lost fat and collagen. They are absolutely amazed by the results after only a short period of time. The beauty of Facercise is that you can create a much more balanced, softened, feminine look to an aging face, and those results can be built upon over weeks, months and years. The possibilities are endless.

What About Botox?

Whether you like it or not, Botox, or Botox Cosmetic as it is often referred to, is a drug. In fact, the Botox Cosmetic website has a long list of possible side effects that look very similar to the multiple symptoms listed in the leaflets accompanying medication we might be prescribed by our doctors, or sold over the counter by the pharmacist. Some of the symptoms on the Botox long list include: problems swallowing, speaking or breathing. It then states: "These problems can happen hours to weeks after an injection of Botox or Botox Cosmetics. Swallowing problems may last for several months. People who cannot swallow well may need a feeding tube to receive food and water." If that's not bad enough, the site goes on to explain the spread of toxin effects. "In some cases, the effect of botulinum toxin may affect areas of the body away from the injection site and cause symptoms of a serious condition called botulism." And if you still aren't convinced, you may like to know that the Botox website lists some "additional inconveniences," including:

- Loss of strength and muscle weakness all over the body
- Double vision
- Blurred vision and drooping eyelids
- Hoarseness or change or loss of voice (dysphonia)
- Trouble saying words clearly (dysarthria)
- Loss of bladder control
- Trouble breathing
- Trouble swallowing

It concludes with the following statement: "Therefore, the long-term effects from using this substance are not really well known or documented." Well, that's all I need to know! I have often wondered about the link between Botox and various autoimmune diseases. The fact remains that we just don't know enough about it.

Many of my clients have reported experiencing bad headaches while using Botox. Some have also experienced a droopy eyelid or eyebrow. Drooping typically occurs when too much Botox is injected into one place or when Botox is injected too close to the eyebrow or eyelid. Others who have used it long term have found that once they stopped using it, their brows sagged and lines formed above the brow.

Injectable Fillers

Injectable fillers come with their own set of problems, including the formation of scar tissue, particularly when it is injected along the nasolabial fold (the two skinfolds that run from each side of the nose to the corners of the mouth; in other words, smile or laugh lines) or the upper lipline. Many clients have come to me in distress over fillers they've had injected into these areas of their face, which are, of course, popular injection sites.

HOW TO BREAK DOWN SCAR TISSUE

Luckily, in my spa I've been able to teach my clients to break down the scar tissue using massage. First, I have them make a long "O" with their mouth. Next, I have them place their index finger along the nasolabial line *inside* their mouth. Using their thumb directly on the nasolabial line *outside* on the skin, I get them to make small circular massaging movements along the entire line to break down the scar tissue. Then I have them perform the same technique along the upper lipline.

Clients are then encouraged to practice the Nasolabial Plumper exercise (see page 74) and/or the Lip Plumper exercise (see page 72) three times a day. This massage technique, along with the exercises, helps many of them restore their faces to normal.

Face the Facts – We're All Aging

Some people are blessed with good genes and age well. Others are not so lucky. It's one thing to be disadvantaged by your genes; however, it's quite another when those fortunate to have *good* genes effectively sabotage that good fortune and accelerate the aging process through overexposure to the sun, smoking, excessive drinking, poor diet, lack of exercise and all sorts of other unhealthy lifestyle factors. However, one very basic fact remains intrinsically stuck in the equation: We cannot stop the inexorable journey that our non-genetic parents – Father Time and Mother Nature – have on our body's aging process. But, we can dramatically slow the impact of their lifelong trek without the use of plastic surgery, Botox, fillers, chemical peels or the like.

The good news is that some of the damage can be reversed by using my facial exercises alongside quality skincare products. The facial exercises will work to build the underlying muscles of your face, and building muscles underneath the skin should help to replace some of the lost fat and collagen and make up for lost volume. This is a process that can be built upon over weeks, months and years, as you continue to exercise your face. Remember, we can't help getting older, but we don't have to *look* older. Toning muscles will lift the skin because the muscles of the face are *attached* to the skin, and don't forget that plumping the muscles under the skin can help erase fine lines and wrinkles as well.

Tightening Your Jawline

A slack jawline – as well as what many refer to as "turkey gobbler neck" or sag underneath the chin and jawline – are common complaints. Performing the Neck Toner (see page 76), the Neck and Chin Lift (see page 82) and the Jaw Toner (see page 78) exercises twice daily will effectively tone the entire neck and jawline, and reduce lines, folds and sag considerably. On the next page is a close-up example of one of my clients, Sharon Martin, who successfully toned her entire neck and jawline. In the first picture, you can see that she had developed a turkey gobbler neck, or what she liked to call

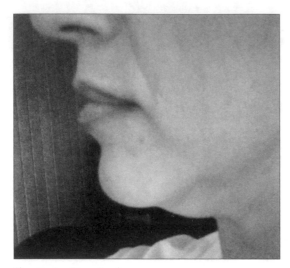

Sharon, pre-Facercise days

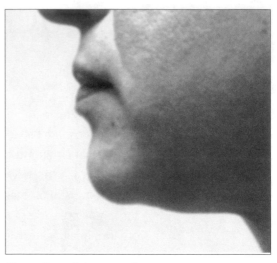

Sharon, "a work in progress"

her "dangling participle." Then, in the second photo, you can see she's made tremendous strides in toning the area beneath her chin. The skin no longer appears loose and dangly. She has firmed and lifted her entire jawline. Sharon herself claims that, "My face *is changing* and looking more and more like it used to before gravity slapped me in the face, literally!" She considers herself "a work in progress," but her results are truly amazing and inspiring. As she continues to Facercise each and every day, she can expect to see some positive changes occur as the weeks, months and years go by. You can see her letter and more photos on page 116.

THE UNWELCOME SIGNS OF AGING
- The skin looks pale, dry and lifeless
- The eyebrows become lower and the eyelids become hooded
- Under-eye puffiness and hollows start to form
- The nose loses its tone and the tip begins to flatten and lengthen
- The lips lose collagen and appear thin and tense-looking
- Lines begin to form above and below the lips
- The corners of the mouth begin to turn down
- Nasolabial lines appear and deepen
- The jawline appears slack and jowls begin to form
- Double chins or loose skin beneath the chin develop
- The neck skin thins and becomes crepey and saggy

THE ULTIMATE REWARDS OF FACERCISE

- The skin awakens and becomes luminous and rosy or peachy-pink
- The eyebrows and lids are lifted and the eyes appear larger and more twinkly
- Under-eye puffiness and hollows diminish
- The nose becomes toned and more perky, the tip lifted and narrowed
- The lips become plump and pink
- Lines begin to diminish around the lips
- Mouth corners are lifted and turn up
- Nasolabial lines soften and diminish
- The jawline firms and appears youthful again
- Double chins and loose neck skin become toned and taut
- The neck skin becomes toned, smoothed and tightened

Other Reasons to Facercise

The benefits of exercising your face daily are numerous for anyone simply dealing with the natural aging process, but it can help others, too. Even young people can have a face that is flatter than it should be, as a result of poor muscle tone, and many have benefited from using my program to make positive changes to their faces. While their skin may be in good condition because they are younger, some young people may have features that they find unappealing. Many young people have written to me to say that they've managed to change a too wide or too narrow face, narrow or shorten their nose, and even plump their lips using Facercise.

What's more, some of my clients have reported suffering from the symptoms of temporomandibular joint syndrome (TMJ). Using the Jaw Toner exercise (see page 78) will help to strengthen and tone the muscles of the jaw to alleviate the pain and muscle soreness from this condition. For others who have dealt with issues such as Bell's palsy, sagging facial muscles due to facial paralysis from stroke, disfigured faces from car accidents, botched plastic surgery, scar tissue from fillers and eyebrow droop after ending Botox treatments, Facercise can be a godsend. I have received many cards and letters over the years from clients who were grateful to have found my program. With Facercise, many of them have been able to gain control over their facial muscles and, as a result, improved their muscle strength, experienced more elastic and firmer skin, and noticed a significant decrease in facial sagging. All of the cards and letters I receive continue to affirm that Facercise can and does work wonders for many different situations – aging being only one of them.

Dear Carole,

I felt compelled to write to you after viewing a video on the Internet made by a doctor who made negative comments about facial exercises. I am by no means an expert in facial exercises, since I have only been doing them for about six months or so, but I do feel that I have a unique perspective on this topic and would like to share my story.

At age 37, nine months after the birth of my first child, I suffered from facial palsy. The entire right side of my face was paralyzed. I had some muscle control because I could blink and did not have slurred speech, but only half of my mouth would smile and my face was drooping from the paralysis. Through treatment, I did regain at least 95 percent of my facial control, but I never really felt like I looked like myself. A few years later while shopping on Amazon I discovered your book, *Facercise*. I was intrigued so I bought the book and the *Beginner Facercise* DVD. The exercises were difficult for me at first because of the facial palsy. Although my face looked almost as it did before, my muscles were so weak!

I couldn't believe the new feeling of circulation I had in my face. Before Facercise, I had slight numbness on the previously paralyzed side of my face, and it disappeared after about a month. Not only was my face starting to look like it did pre-Bell's palsy, but I was starting to look more refreshed and rejuvenated. The amazing thing is that when I laughed or made pretty much any expression after I started Facercise, I could really feel it, like the muscles had been awakened in my face! I had no idea how lifeless my face felt until I started facial exercising. I know it sounds silly but I was able to whistle really well because of my lip strength! Because I was achieving such wonderful results, I wanted to take it a step farther and that's when I scheduled the one-on-one Skype class with you. I have to say that you are gorgeous and youthful-looking! You don't seem to have a line on your face and I cannot believe you are 64!

Carole, your Facercise program has changed my life. I not only have regained the feeling and strength in my face that I lost, but I am looking younger and more vibrant than I have in a long time. Regardless of the claims in the video, I have seen you, and in my mind you are living proof that your facial exercise program does not cause skin damage and sagging if continued for an extended period of time.

Sincerely,
Georgia Tupperman
Atlanta, Georgia

• •

Dear Carole,

A number of years ago I explored other facial exercise programs, but felt they all paled in comparison to your Facercise program. I have been using your program for about six years now. The results are simply amazing. However, I recently got derailed from the program. You see, I was going through loss (death of a loved one), and self care wasn't on my radar. When I "came up for air" and looked in the mirror, I was stunned. I looked years older and absolutely awful. I looked sore and sort of wooden. Ugh! I guess I took for granted what Facercise had done for me and didn't realize the harsh reality until I finally looked in the mirror.

The shocking difference it made to stop doing Facercise for six months last year was very enlightening to say the least. Thankfully, your new Ultimate Facercise program came just in time. So, I'm back on the horse, doing Facercise morning and night. I can already see some positive changes immediately (getting back my glow, smooth tone, contours, etc.). I've developed an eye for subtle changes from listening to you and practicing for so long. Those subtle changes keep me encouraged and motivated. I also know that the cumulative effect will kick in — as it has over the years. I am committed now to keep on doing Facercise daily, nightly and yearly.

You've done your homework, Carole. You're astute and very, very experienced. You understand body systems (skeletal, muscular, endocrine, circulatory, etc.). Lots of wisdom. We are all so very fortunate to have you so actively contributing to the field. I cannot thank you enough.

Mary Ellen Gower
Pawtucket, Rhode Island

Answering the Critics of Facial Exercising

First of all, I'd like to address the various naysayers who unequivocally state that facial exercises do not work and that they are more harmful than beneficial for the skin of the face and the underlying muscles. Some have gone to great lengths to discredit all facial exercise programs. One person even created a special video message on a website proclaiming his personal opinion that facial exercises are not advisable under any conditions.

Bear in mind that these opinions are *not* based on any specific dermatological studies or research. They are not based on science or the educated opinions of some famous doctors, such as Dr. Oz and Dr. Perricone, who both state that facial exercises are good for the face. Nope. It's just based on some naysayers' personal opinions.

OK, enough said. Personally, I put positive results far above personal opinions. Seeing is believing, and that should be enough to convince any doubting Thomas out there.

If you look at a person who exercises regularly, particularly someone who uses weights for resistance training, you'll notice their skin is more toned and taut due to the increased size of the muscles beneath the skin. If you take someone like me, who regularly exercises her face each day and has been doing so for well over 25 years, do you see a wrinkled face? No, quite the opposite.

The very fact that my program has grown, thrived and continued to be successful for myriad people since 1981 is a true testimony to the safety and efficacy of facial exercise. I feel it is fairly safe to assume that muscle-building does not affect the surface of the skin in *any* negative way.

One of the original proponents of bodybuilding was Jack LaLanne. Back in the 1930s, Jack introduced the concept of bodybuilding to the United States. For over ten years, Jack fought with the American Medical

Association (AMA), who tried to run him out of Dodge, claiming that exercise brought on disease such as heart attack and stroke. They tried to discredit his technique and ruin his reputation as an icon in the bodybuilding arena. All the while, Jack persisted, ultimately opening 300 gyms nationwide and continuing to spread the good news that exercise was the key to health and well-being.

At that same time, Jack had developed his own facial exercise program called Face-A-Tonics, which he continued to use and teach even at the ripe old age of 96. His face never suffered from all of the "wear and tear" of exercising.

Jack was an advocate and expert on diet, exercise and nutrition for well over 70 years. He not only talked the talk, but walked the walk. He believed that living a long healthy life is possible by adhering to a healthy diet and healthy lifestyle habits, which include exercising your body and your face. To quote the Godfather of Fitness himself:

"Exercise is king, nutrition is queen; put them together and you have a kingdom!"

Jack also believed that you have to have goals and challenges in life and has been quoted as saying, "Anything in life is possible if you make it happen." I'd like to think that we would all aspire to adopt the same positive thinking as Jack. I know I certainly do.

Facial Exercises *Support,* Not Destroy the Skin

Let's examine the suggestion that stretching out your facial skin results in premature failure of the elastic fibers, causing the skin to sag and stretch out sooner. This has to be one of the most ridiculous statements I have ever heard. Where is the research to back it up? I find it interesting that anyone, whether schooled in the epidemiology of the skin or not, would decide to blame facial exercises for the ultimate destruction of the skin. I would venture a guess that given the current state of the economy, an enlightened public has become more aware of the many benefits of facial exercise. Many of these patients have stopped going in for chemical peels, fillers or Botox. Plenty more have stopped emptying their pocketbooks on expensive creams that promise miracles.

The truth is that Facercise is something that doesn't cost you thousands of dollars, doesn't require any gadgets and works with what God has given you. That's not very good news for the plastic-surgery business – or the manufacturers of beauty products.

Research conducted by the Lancôme Marketing Research Group has determined that people make somewhere in the neighborhood of 15,000 facial movements in a single day. Many of these movements happen to occur while we are speaking, yawning, straining and exercising. That is the equivalent of 450,000 movements a month and over 5,400,000 movements a year. For argument's sake, let's say that the average person lives to be approximately 75 years old. Those of us who live to age 75 will have made the equivalent of around 410,625,000 facial movements in the span of our lifetime. Now that's an awful lot of facial movements. If we were to follow the logic of the naysayers, this number of facial movements would ensure that our skin, having been broken and battered by that point in time, would look much like a crumpled, wrinkled-up piece of paper thrown into the trash can.

Everyday facial movements are *not* to blame for facial wrinkling. One of the main factors contributing to facial lines and wrinkles is overexposure to the sun's harmful rays – and the subsequent breakdown of the collagen, fat and elastin beneath the skin. Furthermore, poor dietary habits, lack of proper hydration and compression of the skin by sleeping with your face scrunched into the pillow all night can eventually wreak havoc on your skin.

I can assure you, however, that the movements you make by moving and exercising your face are not the cause of lines and wrinkles. What's more, exercising your face will make you more aware of the expression lines you are causing by constantly squinting or furrowing your brow to form what I like to call the "question mark" between the brows. All of these can be eased and smoothed with the help of facial exercise.

All of the many cards, letters and emails I receive every day assure me that Facercise is most definitely working for my clients. So why is it that we need research to explain why facial exercises work any more than body exercises do? Muscles are muscles, and each and every one of them can be exercised to grow stronger, firmer and larger. Furthermore, exercising muscles will not stretch them – or your skin – out of shape. The reason that facial exercises do not cause lines to form is simple: With the Facercise program, you are using your hands on your face to stabilize the skin to prevent lines and creases from forming while you work your facial muscles. You are also holding your face in certain positions that will not stretch the skin, and will target and work the muscles correctly. Facial exercises are intended to allow you to move your face naturally, but make you more keenly aware of repetitive facial movements that may become problematic, such as habitual squinting. As you become more "facial aware," bad habits such as squinting or frowning are greatly diminished.

Unfortunately we cannot replace lost collagen and fat beneath the skin, but we can build muscle to compensate for their loss. In fact, exercising your face is as healthy for your skin as exercising is for your body.

Forehead and nasolabial lines can most definitely be plumped up and softened by facial exercises. By building the underlying muscles, lines are eased and the skin is lifted. You also initiate a strong blood supply to the skin, creating a more vibrant complexion and a youthful rosy skin color. Skin becomes more luminous and alive.

Well, that's enough on the naysayers. As I've said in my previous books, critics of Facercise remind me of gongs at level crossings: immovable but still clanging loudly and vainly as the big freight trains roll by.

Medical Professionals Who Support Facial Exercising

The good news is there are plenty of enlightened doctors, dermatologists and dentists who support the benefits of facial exercising. During a recent *Ask Dr. Oz* segment of his popular television show, Dr. Oz was asked to comment on facial exercises – in particular, Facercise. One woman in the studio audience stood and talked about her worries about recently turning 40. She stated that her "appearance anxiety" had gone off the charts and so she bought a book on Facercising.

Dr. Oz asked, "Facercising?"

She replied, "Yes, exercises that are supposed to help you avoid plastic surgery because I'm vain, but I'm cheap."

She explained that she'd been diligently performing the exercises in her bathroom so that her boyfriend wouldn't see her. She seemed a little embarrassed about performing the exercises, but she wanted to know whether they were a "complete and ridiculous waste of her time" or whether they might actually have a positive impact on her appearance. She went on to explain the exercises, saying that they were "resistance-type" exercises. Then she stood up and gave Dr. Oz a demonstration of my Cheek Energizer exercise (see page 66) on national television.

Dr. Oz thoughtfully answered her. "Here's the deal with Facercising. One of the reasons our face muscles sag is because, over time, we begin to lose some of the collagen, the wiring that holds together the muscles in the skin. As it turns out, the Japanese do a lot of Facercising and they have very few wrinkles." (How did he know my books were so popular in Japan?)

He went on to say that, "Pulling out and forcing the muscles back in [resistance exercises] should probably keep those muscles taut and prevent some of the sagging that occurs with gravity," and he ended with the following statement: "It's a pretty straightforward, very rational thing to do, and doesn't cost you any money. I must say that if I were in your shoes, I'd keep doing it."

So there you have it. Keep Facercising. Doctor's orders!

U.S. dermatologist Dr. Nicholas Perricone shares Dr. Oz's viewpoint regarding facial exercises. In his blog, *MD Perricone*, he states, "If your skin has already begun to lose its tone and elasticity, natural facelift options are available." Dr. Perricone also asserts that there are several ways to firm up your skin and that some of the best ways involve natural remedies, such as proper diet and nutrition, taking supplements and getting plenty of exercise. But Dr. Perricone isn't only referring to working the muscles of your body.

He writes, "Exercise is one of the most important practices to maintain for firming your skin. Exercise will help circulation which ultimately results in skin remaining firm and toned." Dr. Perricone sums it up succinctly by stating, "Simple facial exercises are great for tightening the skin of the face."

It's taken some time, but eventually many from the medical establishment have realized the importance of the alternative methods available to help us in our quest to remain youthful. Facercise has continued to grow and flourish across the globe. Countless women and men have been able to firm up their faces and diminish fine lines and wrinkles by using my program. I know many actors and actresses who have decided to abandon Botox because it doesn't allow them freedom of expression while performing. They rely on their facial muscles to be able to express themselves, and with Botox they cannot use their faces the way they would like. Therefore, many of them have opted to use my Facercise program to remain toned, taut and youthful-looking, yet still able to perform. Now it's more important than ever as high-definition TV reveals a lot more than normal TV ever did. As people become better informed, they are making more positive decisions for their overall health and well-being, which includes exercising not only their bodies but their faces, too.

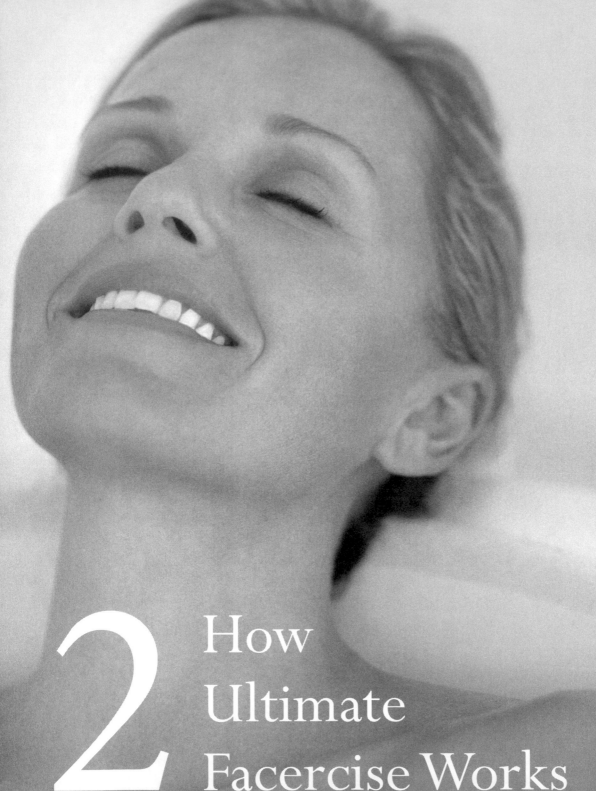

2

How
Ultimate
Facercise Works

If you think about it, exercising your face could be the single most important thing you do to help you return your face to a more luminous and youthful look. Using the Ultimate Facercise program, you will be investing just 16 minutes a day and, ultimately, your face – and your mirror – will thank you. The huge dividends it pays far exceed the small investment of time.

Ultimate Facercise works the muscles of the face and neck in much the same way as my original program, in that it concentrates on the same muscle groups. There are 57 muscles in the face and neck, and all of them work together synergistically to create balance, symmetry and lift. The difference is in the intensity of the program, and the way you use your body differently to achieve more dramatic improvements in a much shorter period of time.

To help you understand how facial exercises work, it's important to understand where the different muscles of the face are located and what their specific functions are. Understanding where the muscles are located as well as the functions they perform will help you to better isolate them while performing the exercises. Many people think because we use our faces to make expressions, we are exercising our muscles in the process. But this is not the case at all. The muscles of the face need to be properly exercised through facial exercise that utilizes resistance in order to remain toned and to become stronger and larger. Resistance can be using your hands on your face – or even through body posturing movements – to create more burn. When you exercise the muscles of the face to the point of exhaustion and can feel the lactic-acid burn, the muscles then need to rest. It is during the rest period that the muscles will be able to recover and then grow. This is a process that can be built upon over the weeks, months and years as you continue to Facercise.

The Ultimate Facercise program contains 13 synergistic exercises. We begin with the eye area and work our way down the face to the neck and jaw area. The reason we don't skip around is because we want to exercise one muscle group to the point of exhaustion and then move on to the next group. Therefore, it is important to follow the program exactly as it was intended.

Live the Dream

Part of the battle with any exercise program is finding the willpower to stick to it, even if you're busy or tired. Before you start, read this section. And come back to it if you feel like giving up.

See It

Take the time to think about what it will feel like to reach your goal with Ultimate Facercise. Then write down all of the changes you would like to see in your face. The first step to creating the face of your dreams is envisioning it. Make it great!

Trust in the Program

Follow the program closely. This program is tried and tested, and designed to work for everyone, so don't fight it. Although the steps are easy, not everyone is ready and willing to trust that it will work. Accept the fact, and then just let the program work its magic. It won't be long before you see results.

Say It Like It Is

Instead of saying, "I can look like this" or "I will look like that," which are simply wishes out there in the future, tell yourself, "I am in control and I am already looking better." By doing this, you are recognizing the positive, subtle changes that are taking place day by day, week by week and month by month. By using the present tense, your brain accepts your words as the ultimate truth.

Take a look at what 30 days of Facercising on a consistent basis can achieve:

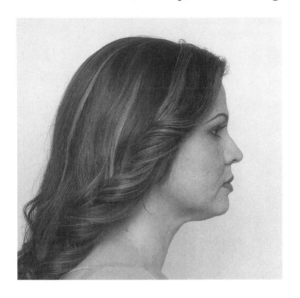 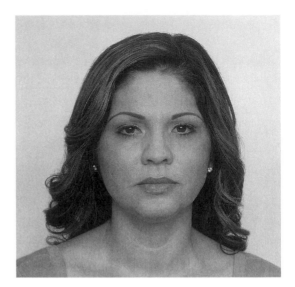

First day: Judith, 36, exhibits an overall lack of muscle tone and a dull complexion. She has drooping eyelids, under-eye puffiness, deep nasolabial folds and a slack jawline.

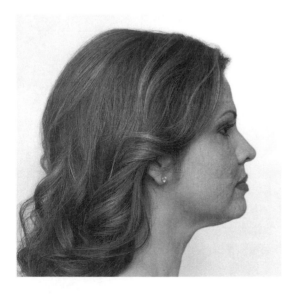 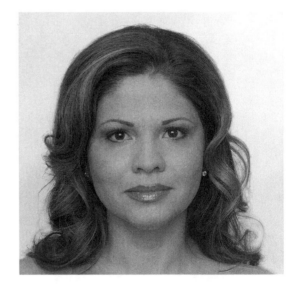

After 30 days: Judith's entire face has a more toned, firmer appearance. Her complexion is vibrant and rosy. Her eyes are more open and youthful-looking. Her under-eye puffiness has diminished, her nasolabial lines are smoother and her jawline is more toned.

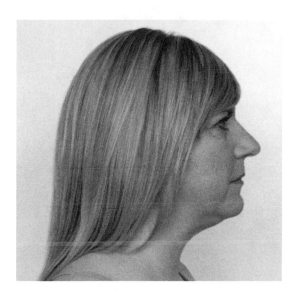
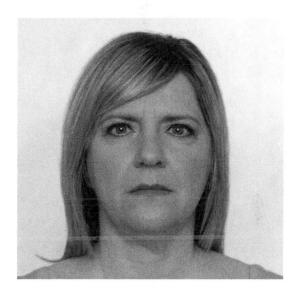

First day. Loree, 51, has a puffy face and an overall lack of tone. Her eyebrows are low on her face and her question-mark lines are pronounced. Her cheeks are flat on her face and she has a heavy jawline.

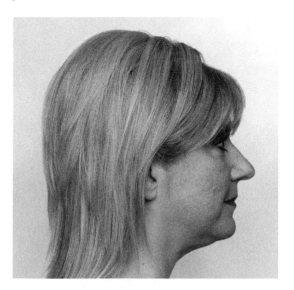
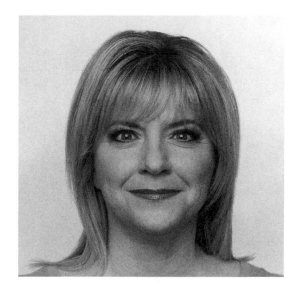

After 30 days: Loree's overall face looks toned and sculpted. Her eyes are more open and brighter. Her brows are higher and the question-mark lines are less apparent. Her cheeks are more full and her chin, neck and jawline are firmer.

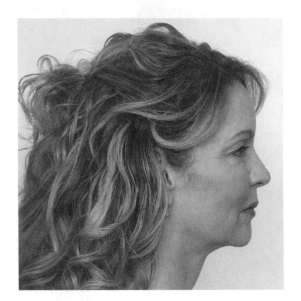 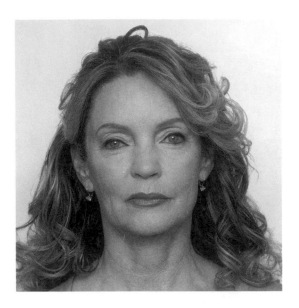

First day: Nancy, 57, has an overall stressed appearance. Her eyes have a tired look. Her cheeks are low and flat on her face. Her jawline has a weak appearance. Her lips are thin and the corners of her mouth are turned down.

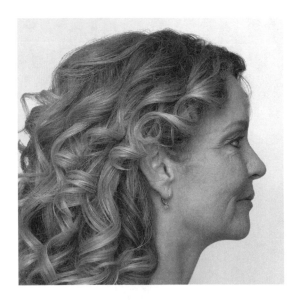 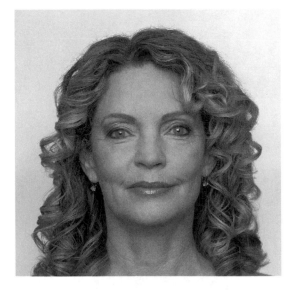

After 7 days: Nancy has a much softer, more youthful appearance. Her eyes are brighter and more open. Her cheeks are higher and fuller. Her lips have plumped up and her jawline is stronger. All this in **seven** days.

Understanding Muscle Groups

Understanding the different muscle groups, where they are located and their specific functions will help you achieve success with the Ultimate Facercise program.

Muscles of the Eye

The eyes are one of the first areas of the face to lose tone and definition. Sometimes even younger people can have droopy upper eyelids due to an inherited trait, which can make them look and appear sleepy-eyed or tired and older than their years. With age, the eyebrows eventually drop, falling into the upper eyelid space and causing the eyes to appear much smaller. Crow's feet start to form at the outer-eye corners and loose skin beneath the eyes will form bags. Other times, there will be a hollowed-out look beneath the eyes, which also makes a person appear old, tired and brittle.

When we open and close our eyes or when we blink, we are engaging the muscle that surrounds the orbit of the eye called the *orbicularis oculi*. However, because muscles don't get stronger by themselves, we won't achieve muscle tone unless we use the muscle against resistance.

The Eye Opener exercise (see page 62) engages the *orbicularis oculi* as well as the *levator palpebrae superioris* muscle, which is a thin muscle located in the upper eyelid. This exercise increases blood flow to the entire area, resulting in brighter, more refreshed-looking eyes. Toning these muscles will reduce crow's feet and give you that eyes-wide-open look. Many of my clients have said this exercise also helps to reduce or eliminate dark under-eye circles. This is because we are flushing toxins from the area. Another exercise that engages the *orbicularis oculi* is the Lower Eyelid Lifter exercise (see page 64), which helps to diminish under-eye hollows and puffiness.

A main contributor to aging eyes is the loss of tone of the *epicranius* muscle. As this muscle begins to lose tone, the eyebrows eventually sag down into the upper eye area, which leads to droopy upper eyelids, resulting in sleepy, tired-looking eyes. The *epicranius* muscle, which allows you to raise up your eyebrows, is a very important muscle to strengthen and tone. Your brows will appear more arched and higher on your face, giving you a more alert look. Your upper eyelids will be toned and firm, and the entire eye area will open up. Performing the Furrow Smoother exercise (see page 63) will strengthen and tone the entire forehead area and pull your eyebrows up higher on your face. It can also help to reduce forehead lines and creases, and create a much more relaxed look.

Muscles of the Scalp

There are numerous muscles located directly beneath the scalp that enable us to raise our eyebrows or to frown. One of these muscles is the *frontalis*, which is part of the *epicranius*, located above the forehead. This muscle is mainly used for frowning, but when engaged during the Furrow Smoother exercise (see page 63), it helps you lift your eyebrows up.

Another muscle, the *occipitalis*, is also part of the *epicranius* and is located at the back of the head. It helps to draw the scalp backwards.

The *galea aponeurotica* is a tendon that covers the upper portion of the scalp and joins the *frontalis* and *occipitalis* muscles. All of these muscles work together synergistically to lift up the eyebrows while performing the Furrow Smoother.

Muscles of the Nose

I have long maintained that the nose continues to grow throughout our entire lives. The reason for this phenomenon is simply a lack of good muscle tone. As the underlying muscles become weak and slack, the tip of the nose widens and turns downward. Much of the nose is comprised of cartilage and muscle, and for this reason the nose can be refined and in some cases even reshaped. Nothing short of a rhinoplasty can actually remove a bump, but exercising the nose tones the muscles, which softens the appearance of the bump.

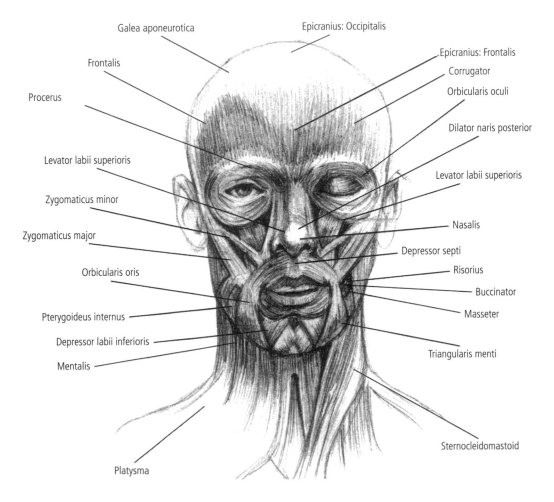

Galea aponeurotica

Frontalis

Procerus

Levator labii superioris

Zygomaticus minor

Zygomaticus major

Orbicularis oris

Pterygoideus internus

Depressor labii inferioris

Mentalis

Platysma

Epicranius: Occipitalis

Epicranius: Frontalis

Corrugator

Orbicularis oculi

Dilator naris posterior

Levator labii superioris

Nasalis

Depressor septi

Risorius

Buccinator

Masseter

Triangularis menti

Sternocleidomastoid

I have had numerous clients tell me that people have asked them if they have had a nose job after they had been doing my Nose Transformer exercise (see page 68) for a while.

Performing the Nose Transformer will effectively shorten and narrow a too wide or long nose. There is even a special variation to help straighten a crooked nose or a nose that curves to one side of the face. We are not talking about *removing* the bump, just straightening a nose that curves to one side. Many of my clients have had great success straightening their noses using this new technique.

There are five muscles in the nose that work together to perform different functions. The first is the *procerus* muscle, which crosses the bridge of the nose and works to pull the middle of the brows in a downward fashion. The *nasalis* starts at the bridge and extends upward, allowing us to compress our nostrils. The *depressor septi* extends across the base of the nose and helps to close the nasal openings by pulling down the septum (the cartilage area between the nostrils).

The *dilatator naris posterior* muscle, which lies near the margin of the nostril, helps us open the nasal passages to allow more air into our lungs, while the *dilatator naris anterior* muscle, which is a thin muscle above the middle of each nostril, helps us to flare our nostrils. All of these muscles can be toned, tightened and lifted by the Nose Transformer.

Muscles of the Ear

The ear has three small muscles that surround it, and they sit directly beneath the surface of the skin. Some people actually have such good control over these muscles that they can effectively wiggle and raise up their ears quite easily. While these muscles are not overly important to the appearance of the face, they do help in various ways when you are performing a number of the facial exercises. The reason for this is that they are connected to other muscles. Remember, this is a synergistic program and all of your muscles count, whether they directly affect your appearance or not. For example, when you are performing the Eye Opener and Furrow Smoother exercises (see pages 62 and 63), you will notice that your ears become engaged. Concentrate on the muscles and flex your ears while you squeeze your eyes shut tight and lift up your brows. This will increase the effectiveness of the exercises.

The first muscle of your ear is the *anterior auricularis*. This small, thin, fan-shaped muscle helps to draw the ear forward. When you are performing the Jaw Toner exercise (see page 78), you might even notice that your ears flex ever so slightly. Again, this is because all of the muscles are interconnected at various points on the face.

The *superior auricularis* is the next muscle that helps you lift the ears upward. You may not even feel this muscle move or play any specific role, but it is working hard while you perform the Face Contour exercise (see page 80). Using the mind–muscle connection while you visualize the sides of your face lifting can have a tremendous impact on the results you achieve while performing this exercise. Imagine not only the sides of your face lifting, but your ears as well.

The *posterior auricularis* draws the ears backward. If you use your mind–muscle connection while performing the Face Filler (see page 65), think of pushing your ears back and expanding your cheeks out. This will help you widen and fill in that gaunt area of your lower face.

Muscles of the Mouth

Many women automatically think they need to use cosmetic fillers such as fat, collagen or Restylane to plump their lips. Others will take a more drastic route and have their lips enhanced with permanent implants. Although the fillers will temporarily plump the lips, they cannot restore the mouth corners to their youthful, upturned position and neither will permanent implants. But there is another solution for the lips. The Lip Lift and Lip Plumper exercises (see pages 70 and 72) will absolutely refine, reshape and plump your lips. There are many muscles of the mouth and the surrounding areas that will be affected by the Lip Plumper, Lip Lift, Cheek Energizer and Face Contour exercises.

The *orbicularis oris* completely surrounds the mouth and its muscular fibers connect with other fibers in the upper and lower lips, cheeks, nose and surrounding areas. This muscle allows you to close your lips. When you perform the Lip Plumper and Cheek Energizer (see pages 72 and 66) you will feel this muscle become engaged and eventually become toned.

The *buccinator* is a thin, broad muscle located at each side of the face underneath the cheek, and it assists in the act of sucking. While performing the Cheek Energizer and Face Contour (see pages 66 and 80) you will effectively tone, strengthen and build this muscle.

The *triangularis menti* is a triangular muscle that extends from the lower jaw up to the mouth.

It is responsible for drawing your mouth corners down when you pout. By performing the Lip Lift twice daily, you will tone and turn up the corners of your mouth.

Moving on, the *risorius* muscle is a band of fibers that help when you smile, and the Lip Lift will also tone this muscle. The *zygomaticus major* and *minor* muscles are used when you laugh, drawing your mouth up and back. These muscles will also be efficiently toned by the Lip Lift exercise.

The *quadratus labii inferioris* is a small quadrilateral muscle that pulls your lower lip down into a small pout. The Lip Plumper will ensure that this muscle remains strong and toned. Lastly, the *caninus* is a small muscle that allows you to raise your upper lip into a sneer. Keeping this muscle toned is easy with the Lip Plumper.

Muscles of Mastication

Having a nicely toned jawline is something that all men and women admire and desire. The jawline usually begins to lose its tone somewhere in your mid to late thirties. But, for those who have spent too much time in the sun, that time may arrive sooner rather than later. As we enter our forties and fifties, we develop jowls. The Jaw Toner exercise (see page 78) will effectively tone, tighten and lift the entire jawline to restore that youthful look to your face. The *masseter* and *temporalis* work in conjunction with each other to close the teeth with force, particularly when you chew food or gum – or if you grind your teeth while sleeping.

The *pterygoideus externus* is a thick, cone-shaped muscle that helps you open your mouth and rotate your jaw, while the *pterygoideus internus* is another muscle that helps you mash and crush your food. Using all of these muscles during the Jaw Toner, you can keep your jawline toned, tightened and lifted.

Muscles of the Neck and Chin

The neck is another major area of concern, particularly for women. As we age, the skin on the neck begins to thin and sag, causing neck rings to form. Sleeping on your side or stomach will make matters worse, as this tends to create additional lines and creases on your neck. A nicely toned neck gives the appearance of youth, something all women (and men) desire.

The *platysma* is a thin broad band of muscular fibers located underneath the skin on either side of the neck. This is a very

powerful muscle that enables you to push down your lower jaw. It becomes engaged while you perform the Jaw Toner (see page 78), and exercising this muscle will smooth and tone the skin of the neck.

The *sternocleidomastoid* is a broad, thick and powerful muscle that is activated when you rotate your head from side to side. The Neck and Chin Lift exercises (see page 82), as well as the Neck Toner (see page 76), work very well to keep this muscle toned and strong.

The *trapezius* is a muscle located at the back of the neck and shoulders. It helps you turn your head from side to side and works in conjunction with the *sternocleidomastoid* muscle. The Neck and Chin Lift and Neck Toner exercises work all of these muscles, keeping the neck long and strong and beautiful.

How to Keep on Track

● ●

Many people question whether facial exercises can actually work to reshape the face. I can answer them with a resounding, "Yes they can. Absolutely!" Done correctly, facial exercises can reshape the face by creating symmetry and balance. They can also create fullness, and lift and diminish fine lines and wrinkles. I have often had to give myself a healthy reality check if I begin to feel doubtful about my own program. The message I am playing in my own head says, "Is it *really* the exercises or something else that I'm doing that

has kept my face looking so good?"

It is during those times that I need to take a break from my exercise regime. Why? Because within a few days I start to notice changes on my own face that I don't particularly like. My face starts to look *tired*. It doesn't appear as toned and taut, and my skin seems less vibrant and luminous. I, of course, immediately return to my routine, and things swing back to normal again. Believe it or not, this little trick actually keeps me focused, motivated and on track with my daily regime.

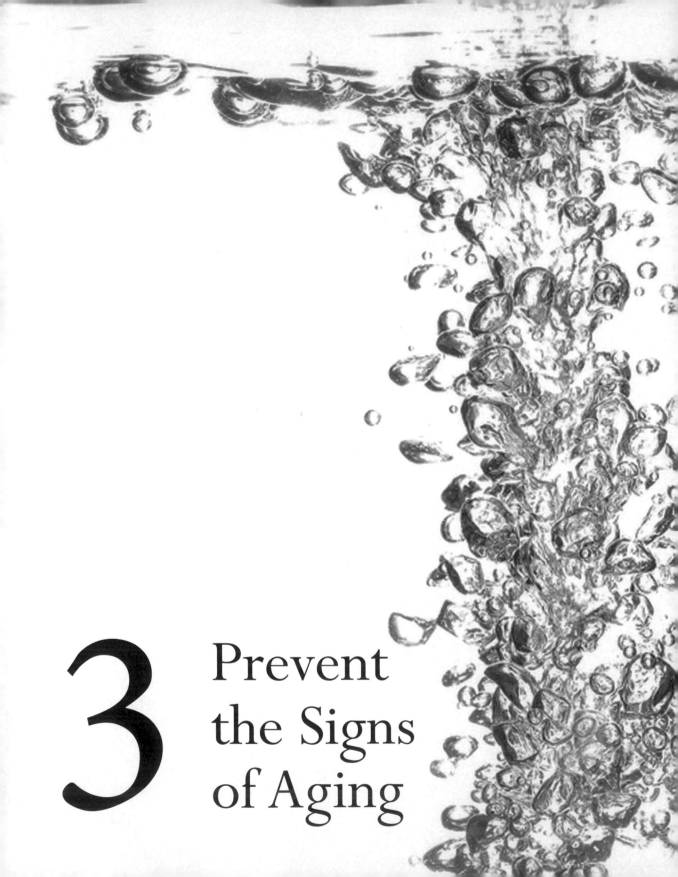

3 Prevent the Signs of Aging

Without a doubt, the Ultimate Facercise program will help you create some truly positive changes in your face. You need to set a course of action, create a goal for yourself, be consistent and stick to the plan. However, in order to be successful with my program, you also need to consider some of the things you may be doing that could actually be aging your face more quickly. More and more studies have shown how poor nutrition, lack of sleep, leading a sedentary lifestyle and excess stress can all wreak havoc on your body. We need to address those issues and fully understand how poor choices can affect our skin and cause it to age prematurely.

Succeeding with Ultimate Facercise

In order to get the most from the Ultimate Facercise program, it's important to adopt some healthy lifestyle changes that will nourish and protect your skin from the inside and out. Not only will this help to turn back the clock and have an impact on your overall health and well-being, but alongside your Facercise exercises, you'll notice a dramatic difference in the face you present to the world.

Getting the Right Diet

As the saying goes, "You are what you eat," and nothing could be closer to the truth. Healthy skin, hair and nails all reflect a healthy body and lifestyle, especially as you age. By middle age, the poor eating habits that you once got away with in your twenties are a path that you can no longer take. Consistently unhealthy dietary choices will start to show up on your face if you don't take good care of yourself.

As you may realize by now, Facercise is more than just a facial exercise program; it's a way of life. Not only is good-quality nutrition important to nourish the body and sustain life, but it enables your body to repair connective tissues, build and repair cells, and maintain healthy, vibrant, luminous skin. For example, a diet lacking in adequate levels of fresh fruits, vegetables, protein and essential fatty acids (EFAs or "omega" oils) can thwart your body's ability to build muscle and to keep the skin soft and supple.

What to Do

Avoid Refined Foods

For many people, refined foods (such as white flours and white rice) are a staple of their diet, but it's been established that excessive amounts of refined foods can actually prematurely age the skin. The reason for this is a natural process known as glycation, in which the sugar in your bloodstream attaches to proteins to form harmful new molecules called advanced glycation end products (or AGEs for short). Many of us have diets that contain too many processed foods, with very high levels of carbohydrates, such as pizza, pasta, bagels, rice, cookies, refined cereals and chips. Refined carbohydrates are converted into sugar by the body; therefore, the more refined foods (sugar) you eat, the more AGEs you will develop.

When selecting packaged carbohydrates such as breads and muffins, avoid brands with labels that read "enriched," "bleached" and "unbleached" – "Semolina," "durum wheat" and "white rice" are also to be avoided. These are most certainly processed grains that have been stripped of their valuable nutrients. The whiter a product, the more likely it is to have been processed, and had the majority of its goodness stripped away.

For example, when white rice is refined, it is milled to remove the husk, bran and germ from the grain. Brown rice is a much healthier choice because, even after the husk is removed, the other layers remain intact. It's been reported that brown rice can stabilize blood sugar levels, help lower high blood pressure and reduce the risk of heart attack, and possibly prevent certain types of cancers.

Whole grains – grains that contain all of the naturally occurring nutrients of the entire grain seed, and have not had anything stripped or removed from them in the manufacturing process – are positively encouraged, because they contain a wealth of nutrients that will nourish your skin and the tissues beneath. So, always look for 100 percent whole grain or whole-wheat versions of carbohydrate foods.

According to Dr. Fredric Brandt, a dermatologist with practices in Miami and New York, "As AGEs accumulate [as a result of eating refined foods], they damage adjacent proteins in a domino-like fashion." Most vulnerable to damage are collagen and elastin, the protein fibers that keep skin firm and elastic.

Furthermore, dermatologist Dr. Nicholas Perricone states, "When our blood sugar goes up rapidly and continually, the sugar can actually attach to the collagen in our skin, making it stiff and inflexible. When your collagen is cross-linked by sugar, you end up with stiff and sagging skin."

If that is not enough, he goes on to say, "When glycation occurs in the skin, the ultimate effect is not unlike tanning a hide. Over time, skin begins to resemble a cross between beef jerky and an old boot, unevenly discolored and heavily striated with deep lines and grooves." That statement alone should be enough to keep your hand out of the cookie jar!

My best advice would be to avoid all carbohydrates after 5 p.m. because they cause overall facial bloat and under-eye puffiness. If you need a snack after 5, opt for cucumber or celery sticks, low-fat string cheese, olives or some slices of avocado. If you eat a well-balanced diet, focusing on whole foods directly from the earth, such as fruits and vegetables, and choose high-quality proteins, you will be protecting your overall health and the health of your skin as well.

Eat Protein

All muscles need protein to build and repair; however, according to Dr. Perricone, "The contemporary American [and, indeed, Western] diet rarely contains protein in sufficient quantity to maintain and repair cell and skin health." The reason for this is not that we don't get plenty of *sources* of protein, but that the sources we choose are not high quality, and therefore have little impact on our health.

Make sure your diet contains two portions of high-quality protein each day. Try to include choices such as chicken, turkey, fish, eggs or lean meats, which are "complete" proteins and most easily used by the body.

Vegetarians also need to make sure to include quality protein choices in their diets to help them repair and build strong muscles. Good options for vegetarians, which will also encourage good overall skin health in meat eaters, include a wide range of pulses (kidney beans, chickpeas, soy and lentils, etc.), unsalted nuts and seeds, and some dairy products. The greater the variety of proteins you have in your diet, the more likely you are to get the nutrients you need.

Watch the Salt

We need to limit our salt intake, too. Salt causes the body to retain water, and too much of it can make you look like a mini Michelin man, not to mention spiking your blood pressure. Even if you don't add salt to your food, chances are that you're ingesting more than you realize by eating fast foods, junk foods or anything that is heavily processed. Check the labels of the foods you eat regularly; salt can even be added to "healthy" foods like breakfast cereals, canned vegetables and bread. It's recommended that an adult consume no more than 6 grams of salt a day (about a teaspoonful), which is the equivalent of 2.4 grams of sodium.

Drink Enough Water

Getting your eight glasses of water each day is another important factor in maintaining a healthy body and keeping your skin radiant and wrinkle-free. But, according to Dr. Perricone, "Most people walk around in a state of mild dehydration at all times." Water is vital to all of our cells, and it is especially important to the health of our skin by increasing elasticity, moisturizing, repairing skin tissue and keeping it looking tight. Muscles are also comprised of 75 percent water and therefore need sufficient water to help them grow and look "full." These are all very good reasons to keep yourself properly hydrated, particularly as you age.

Making poor dietary choices will eventually wreak havoc on your complexion, creating rough skin and wrinkles, and a puffy face that lacks good muscle tone and lift.

You may be surprised to learn that poor diet is probably the biggest reason why many young people look older than their actual age, and it's one thing over which you have *complete* control.

THE ANTI-INFLAMMATORY DIET

Many doctors, such as Dr. Perricone, prescribe an anti-inflammatory dietary approach, which is said to firm the skin and reduce wrinkles. The heart of his diet is very straightforward and can have a positive impact on your health and the health of your skin.

He suggests:

- Wild Alaskan salmon, because it contains high levels of DMAE (a natural chemical that some people call "a facelift in a jar"), astaxanthin (a carotenoid or brightly colored pigment) and essential fatty acids (EFAs, see below), which increase the skin's firmness and create radiance and glow. Astaxanthin is also found in other types of seafood besides salmon, as well as certain marine plants and algae.
- Olive oil is recommended because it contains high levels of oleic acid, which help the cells absorb essential fatty acids. It also contains a high level of quality antioxidants and natural anti-inflammatories known as polyphenols.
- Avocados are also high in oleic acid, a monounsaturated fat, and contain high levels of the antioxidant carotenoid lutein, as well as other carotenoids and significant quantities of tocopherols (vitamin E). Avocados are an excellent choice because they contain high-quality fat and protein, and help the body absorb more fat-soluble nutrients when eaten with other foods.
- Antioxidants are another important component of Dr. Perricone's dietary recommendations as they help slow the aging process, enhance the immune system, and lower your risk of heart disease and cancer. He suggests that blueberries and other dark berries, as well as red and purple grapes, contain high levels of antioxidants that belong to the flavonoid group of phytonutrients, which are of particular interest when it comes to skin health and antiaging. Vegetables that contain flavonoids include beets, kale, red onions, green beans and endive. Carotenoids are also very potent antioxidants that can help slow down the degenerative effects of aging, and are found in brightly colored yellow, orange, red and green vegetables and fruits. The highest carotenoid levels are found in carrots, red bell peppers, tomatoes and green leafy vegetables.

Cruciferous vegetables, such as broccoli, cauliflower, Brussels sprouts and turnips, should also be included in your diet, as they contain some special phytonutrients that protect against certain cancers and enhance the health of your skin.

- Omega oils have been shown to help skin look most youthful, and they have a host of other important benefits in the body, many of which are considered to be antiaging. Omega oils contain fatty acids that moisturize the skin from within, reduce fluid loss from the skin, support the integrity of cell membranes, and provide the skin with the nutrients it needs to maintain optimal health. Great sources are freshwater fish and their oils, nuts, seeds, hemp seeds and oils, and leafy green vegetables.

Supplements

Before you embark on a supplementation program, it is always wise to talk to your doctor to be sure you are taking the right supplements in the correct doses for your body's particular needs. Dr. Oz says to "remember your ABCs," which reminds us to take all-important vitamins A, B and C.

He states, "Vitamin A keeps your skin strong and allows it to create new layers, vitamin B is an important metabolism enhancer and vitamin C rebuilds the collagen at your skin's base."

Personally, I use a high-quality multivitamin supplement in powder form, as well as powdered Ester C, because I feel that powdered products allow for better absorption of the nutrients they contain. I also take various essential fatty acids (EFAs), such as cod liver oil, cold-pressed virgin olive oil and omega-3 oils with DPA and DHA. Another supplement that I have included in my daily regime is an excellent product called Pure Synergy. Pure Synergy, an organic superfood supplement that you mix into water, encourages overall health, energy and well-being. Altogether, these supplements can make up for shortfalls in your diet and encourage the health of your skin, both inside and out.

Natural Hormones

As a full-time owner of a spa, working six days a week, a wife, a mother and a grandmother, I keep myself pretty busy. As you can imagine, I need all the help I can get to keep up with my busy schedule and life. So how exactly do I go about accomplishing all of this?

In my early forties, I started to experience some of the many unpleasant side effects and symptoms of hormonal fluctuations. While I'd been exercising my face since age 36, and felt I looked pretty good for age 40, my energy levels were gradually beginning to wane. Now, I wasn't *feeling* as good as I looked, and I knew I was experiencing perimenopausal symptoms. Around that time, many of my friends were also experiencing some of the same symptoms that I was, and many of them decided to take the traditional hormone replacement therapy (HRT).

I had read about some of the HRT side effects, which included risks I was not willing to chance, and knew somewhere deep inside me that this was not the path I would take. I trusted my gut feelings – something I've done my whole life, and a trait that has helped me so much along my life's journey – and began to look at the alternatives. I vividly remembered a poem by Robert Frost, which I read back in high school, called "The Road Not Taken." Frost wrote that while traveling down a path, he came to a fork in the road he was following and didn't know which he should take. After some thought, he "took the one less traveled by / And that has made all the difference." I decided to do the same thing.

My path started when I decided to seek out a doctor to work with me to balance my hormones. I found one who specialized in natural or bioidentical hormones made from plant sources. These hormones are considered bioidentical because they are exactly the same chemical configuration as the hormones our bodies make. To this day, I continue to use bioidentical hormones.

Dr. Uzzi Reiss, prominent obstetrician/gynecologist and antiaging doctor for many Hollywood stars, states, "I emphasize [to my patients] that these are natural hormones that are precise replicas of their own hormones. I use them to prolong optimal hormonal balance that women have in their twenties and thirties, and the results are magnificent." He goes on to describe natural hormones as your foundation, much like the foundation of a house. If the foundation is crumbling, what is the use of painting the house or remodeling it? I agree wholeheartedly with Dr. Reiss and feel that taking bioidentical hormones is one of the best personal decisions I've made for my overall health and well-being.

The fact of the matter is that we are living longer, so why not live the best life possible? Replacing the hormones we've lost by middle age does many wonderful things for the body, and it also does many wonderful things for the face. Waning estrogen causes a loss of skin radiance, and the skin becomes dry and thin, and wrinkles more easily. The loss of progesterone causes water retention, sleep deprivation, anxiety and an overall lack of balance. And these are just some of the symptoms of low hormone levels. Once I began replacing my hormones with bioidentical hormones, I was back to feeling like my old self again. My body's response to natural hormones was amazing; it was as if my body had given me a thumbs-up and a huge sigh of relief.

Sleep Patterns

In today's society many people are sleep deprived. Studies show that an adult needs a good seven to eight hours a night to function properly. Lack of proper sleep can reflect poorly on your overall health and well-being. It's been linked to stress, obesity and even heart disease. Getting a good night's rest *every* night is essential to our antiaging strategy because our cells undergo continuous repair while we sleep. Have you ever noticed that one of the first places that lack of proper sleep shows up is on the face? Of course you have. Dark circles and bags underneath the eyes accompanied by dull and sagging skin are just some of the signs that you're not getting your required seven to eight hours a night.

According to Dr. Oz, under-eye bags can be either short or long term. He claims that the short-term ones are caused by a lack of sleep and I would have to agree. "If you haven't slept all that long, that means you're probably stressed-out," he says. "You start to swell because your body feels stress. Your ankles swell, and so does the tissue under your eyes." He also goes on to explain how sleep is important for your antiaging regime. He states, "Sleep will also generate growth hormone. That's the vitality hormone that makes us nice and bouncy and youthful and vigorous and 'helps' make us stay beautiful. The best way of getting growth hormone is to sleep the seven hours we speak of." Poor sleeping habits will prematurely age you as well. By this I mean sleeping with your face scrunched up and buried in a pillow all night. I cannot overstate the importance of sleeping on your back in order to avoid "pillow face," and deep etched lines from sleeping with your face buried into the pillow.

When you wake in the morning after sleeping all night in this position, your face will look puffy and swollen and your skin will have been pulled and stretched. After some time, the skin will begin to sag, and eventually the sleep lines you see in the morning will become permanent.

I always tell my clients to sleep on their backs without a pillow – or to use a neckroll instead of a pillow. Moreover, placing pillows under your knees will help keep the spine properly aligned. You can also place a small pillow on your chest to hug and give you a feeling of security – as if you were sleeping in the fetal position. But for some, this is a very difficult task, especially if they were always stomach or side sleepers. Luckily, there are many different types of pillows available on the market today to assist you in this process. There are even some that claim to allow you to sleep on your side without scrunching your face in the pillow. They claim to suspend the face and protect the delicate facial tissue.

Here are just a few of the ones that I am aware of:
- The Harley Designer Face Saver Memory Foam Cushion
- The Save My Face Anti-Wrinkle Pillowette
- The Therapeutica Pillow
- The Beauty Pillow

Many dermatologists agree, including Dr. Katie Rodan, who states, "I can usually tell what side a patient sleeps on when I look at her face. The wrinkles will be more compressed, and they might have an unnatural line next to their nose from the pressure." Dr. Rodan recommends Therapeutica pillows, which cradle your head in bed so you can sleep face-up. There are many choices out there, so choose a good pillow that helps you avoid those nighttime enemies.

Sun Protection

• •

I don't need to tell you that skin damage from UV exposure is cumulative. Even those daily trips running errands, or the drive or walk to and from work, with the sun beating down on your face, is causing damage. When it comes to the sun, you can run but you can't hide. Acccording to Dr. Perricone, "When we walk out into the noonday sun during the summer, within five minutes the sunlight creates free radicals in the skin. This results in an inflammatory cascade that accelerates the aging process, causing wrinkles, pre-cancers and cancer as well as discoloration."

We all know someone who has been a sun worshipper or tanning-salon queen and who suffers from premature sag and wrinkles. Looking like heavily tanned leather or a slab of beef jerky is not attractive, no matter how you look at it. Daily application of SPF 30 sunscreen to all exposed skin is a good habit to get into, to avoid a lot of future damage. Make it part of your daily routine, just like brushing your teeth. Remember, it's a whole lot easier to prevent sun damage than it is to reverse it.

I apply my sunscreen directly after my skincare products. If you are wondering which are the safest ones to use, Dr. Perricone recommends physical sunscreens (also known as sunblocks), which physically block the UV rays and don't get absorbed into the skin. "They are nothing more than tiny little particles made out of zinc or titanium that act as minute mirrors that reflect the sun's rays. Chemical sunscreens, by contrast, work by interacting with the skin cells and absorbing the sun's energy and protecting cells in that manner. I feel physical sunscreens, because they do not interact with the cells, are more desirable." I concur. I personally carry and use a physical sunscreen every single day and, at age 64, I do not have any brown spots on my face, hands or arms.

Protecting your skin against the ravages of the sun's detrimental effects is a very important component to your skincare regime. Always apply sunscreen as your last product, after your skincare preparations (although before applying your makeup). Apply it to your face, your neck, the tops of your hands and your arms. And, when out in the sun, don't forget a good pair of sunglasses. Whether you realize it or not, we all tend to squint in the sun, and good sunglasses help prevent squinting.

Dry-Brushing

I have found that dry-brushing is one of the more important elements I have added to my daily skincare regimen. Many people who dry-brush their skin daily find that it complements their detoxification programs and encourages healthy, glowing skin. The reason for this is that dry-brushing exfoliates and sheds the dead skin cells, allowing the skin to breathe and function better.

You may be wondering why we need to bother doing this when our body sheds skin cells on its own. Here's the answer: While it's true that the skin does a pretty good job of shedding dead skin cells, this process starts to slow down dramatically as we age. As this is happening, the skin starts to look dull and begins to lose its youthful glow, often appearing pale. The exfoliation process initiates a strong blood supply to the skin and the skin takes on a rosy color. Daily dry-brushing effectively accelerates the turnover process, making way for fresh new cells. Dull skin will actually start to become more radiant again! Dry-brushing the face will exfoliate, tone, tighten and lift the skin of the face and neck. It will also encourage your skin to absorb your skincare products more efficiently, making it a win–win process.

I begin my day by dry-brushing my entire body with my Horsehair or Sisal Louffa Mitt, and then doing the same on my face, using my Bamboo Glove, which is gentle enough to be used every day. This practice keeps my face glowing the entire day. In the evenings, after cleansing, I use the Beauty Face Mitt, an exfoliating glove that removes dead skin cells and tightens the skin, and repeat the process.

Your Face and Neck

I recommend 30 small circular movements on each section of the face and neck using the Bamboo Glove in the morning and the Beauty Face Mitt in the evening. The fibers of the Bamboo Glove are rougher on the skin, while the Beauty Face Mitt is made of cotton. However, they both exfoliate the dead skin cells, stimulate circulation, and help tone, tighten and lift the skin of the face and neck. Use strong enough pressure to feel as though you are massaging your skin. I advise my clients to make a long "O" with their mouth, to keep the skin firm, and then make 30 circular motions on each area of their face. You will be amazed how dry-brushing brings renewed color, radiance, glow and tone to your skin. It becomes addictive. You will once again have that youthful glow.

Your body

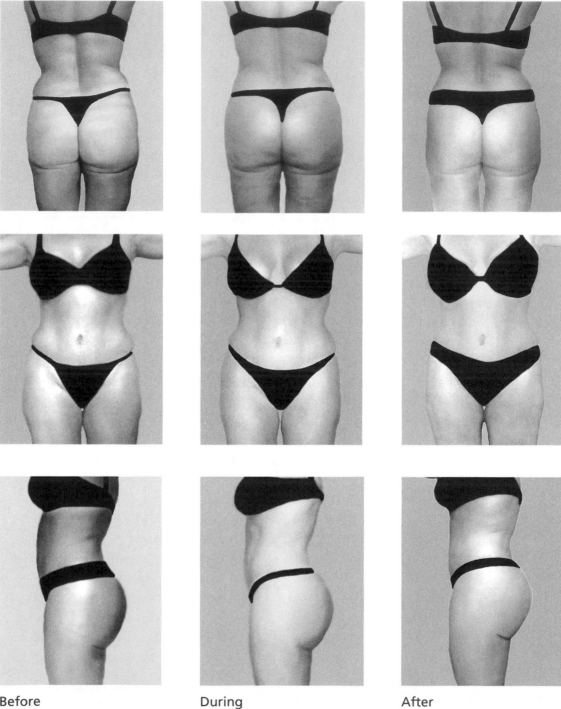

Before   During   After

Dry-brushing your body should also be performed every day to keep your skin looking its best. I recommend and sell a variety of loofahs designed for this purpose. The Sisal Louffa Mitt and Strap are great to start with, because skin that isn't used to dry-brushing might feel sensitive at first. The Sisal Louffa Strap is for addressing the back of your body. I recommend using at least 30 back-and-forth strokes on each area of the body, to strengthen, tone and tighten the skin, break down cellulite deposits, improve muscle tone, stimulate immune function and detoxify the skin. Actually, the more strokes you do, the better your results will be. I personally perform at least 60 to 80 scrubs per area. You should apply strong enough pressure to initiate strong blood supply to the skin, which will make the skin appear pink when you are finished with the process.

Begin by brushing the bottom of the foot from the toes to the heel, then the top of the foot from the toes to the ankle. Next, brush the front and back of the leg from the ankle to the knee, using quick back-and-forth strokes. Proceed to brush from the knee to the top of the front of your thigh – and inner- and outer-thigh areas – using quick back-and-forth strokes, and making certain you cover the entire thigh area. Then repeat the same sequence on the opposite side of your body.

Brush upward strokes over the entire buttock and hip areas. Next, brush up your waistline from hip bones to your natural waist, covering the entire front of your body. Brush the palm of your hand from fingers to the wrist, and repeat on the back of your hand. Brush upward from your wrist to your elbow, front and back. Now brush from elbow to shoulder, front and back. Brush under the bust from the side to the center of your body in semicircular strokes. Brush from the armpit across the top of the bust area, to prevent or eliminate a flabby armpit.

For the back of your body, use the Sisal Louffa Strap. While standing, place the strap at the back of your ankles. Holding the handles, shimmy the strap upward, working your way up to your neck (as if drying yourself with a towel.)

As your skin begins to detoxify, it will become less sensitive and more accustomed to dry-brushing. At this stage, you can then move on to the Horsehair Mitt. The mitt that I use, which is made in Germany, is excellent for creating even more positive changes in the skin. The reason I tell my clients to wait before using this mitt is that it is much rougher on the skin than the Sisal Louffa Mitt. The skin needs to build up a resistance before using this mitt, but the results will be worth the wait.

The Power of Quality Skincare

Never underestimate the power of good-quality skincare products. Working closely with my chemists, I have developed my own line of skincare products. I used to have fine lines and wrinkles due to sun damage and collagen loss in my pre-Facercise days – when I lived in Arizona and baked myself out in the sun, striving for that beautiful tan, and using baby oil and iodine as suntan lotion. Just thinking about that now gives me chills. However, with the help of facial exercises and quality skincare, I have been able to erase virtually all of the visible signs of aging. One thing that I have found over the years is that consistency pays off when it comes to your personal skincare regime. I know that some people say you should never bite off more than you can chew, but the fact is that you simply cannot try something for a short period of time and expect to see fabulous results. That's like standing in front of a microwave oven, frantically shouting, "Hurry up, hurry up." Results from using topical treatments are cumulative.

I also like to alternate products because you cannot possibly include all of the important active ingredients needed for healthy skin in one product. For that reason, my line includes a number of different products and they all serve important roles in antiaging. Old standbys like vitamin C and retinol continue to be utilized in many skincare products, including my own line, because they have been proven to work. Vitamin C, for example, has been found to be very important in hydrating and plumping up the skin, and studies have also shown that it helps build new collagen. Retinol, another favorite of mine for its restorative abilities (without the side effects of Retin-A, which include redness, peeling, sensitivity to sunlight, skin irritation and stinging, as well as severe allergic reactions), is another important weapon to have in your antiaging skincare arsenal.

Newer technologically advanced "actives" found in skincare today, such as epidermal growth factor (EGF) and spin trap (a form of nitrogen antioxidant) are also very important to the overall health and integrity of your skin. EGF works by stimulating cell growth. It is readily available in men's skin;

however, because EGF is androgen dependent, most women don't have enough of it, potentially encouraging the skin to age more quickly. Heavy water (deuterium oxide or D20) is another important active I have included in many of my products. The reason for this is that D20 resists evaporation, dries out more slowly and helps the skin retain moisture. Simply put, moist skin is more youthful-looking skin.

Skincare Staples

Old standbys, such as vitamin C, vitamin E, and retinol, and now spin traps are all very important for the overall integrity and health of the skin and that is why you will continue to find them in many popular skincare preparations. In their recent book, *You Being Beautiful*, Doctors Oz and Roizen recommend the importance of topical agents, retinol (vitamin A), vitamin C and vitamin E to maintain good healthy skin. In his book, *The Wrinkle Cure*, Dr. Perricone recommends spin traps. Let's look at them now:

Vitamin C

In a recent article published in *Life Extension* magazine, vitamin C is touted as a highly important component in the body's production of collagen. In fact, studies have shown that topical application of vitamin C helps boost collagen synthesis and slow its degradation. Also, topical application of vitamin C produces higher concentrations in the skin – apparently 20 times more effectively than oral supplementation. Furthermore, once absorbed in the skin, vitamin C cannot be rubbed or washed off and, even after application has stopped, significant amounts remain in the skin for up to three days. Constant application of vitamin C to the skin rejuvenates its appearance and can help to maintain healthy, younger-looking skin, especially as we age. The article states that vitamin C, especially when combined with green tea extracts, provides even greater skin protection because they both defend the skin against UV exposure and free-radical damage through their antioxidant properties. Doctors Oz and Roizen both recommend topical vitamin C in the form of L-ascorbic acid. This is the most stable form of the vitamin.

Vitamin E

Like vitamin C, vitamin E is a highly effective antioxidant, particularly because it is lipid-soluble (fat-soluble). In a nutshell, this means that it can easily penetrate the skin's surface. In conjunction with water-soluble vitamin

C, vitamin E can effectively protect the skin from free-radical damage. This is the reason you will find vitamin E added to many skincare preparations. Vitamin E is effective when taken orally or applied topically. It seems to protect the skin, particularly from age spots and scarring, and also boosts the skin's natural moisture-retaining properties. According to Doctors Oz and Roizen, topical vitamin E needs to be in the form of D-alpha-tocopherol for the best results. They state that many skin creams contain a form called tocopherol acetate, but confirm that this particular form doesn't help the skin – and, in fact, may even cause some harm. They say, "The real vitamin E stuff [D-alpha-tocopherol] blocks the cancer-causing effects of UV light, stops the immune system from getting blitzed and slows wrinkle production."

Retinol (Topical Vitamin A)

According to Doctors Oz and Roizen, vitamin A wins hands down as the most valuable topical agent when applied to the skin. Why? They state, "Without vitamin A (a 'retinoid'), your skin, hair, and nails will be dry." Vitamin A comes in many forms, such as retinoic acid (Retin-A), retinol, retinaldehyde or retinyl propionate. They claim that all of these forms work because your body can transform one into another and effectively use them all. Topical vitamin A increases stretchy elastin fibers, hardy structural collagen and the natural moisturizer hyaluronic acid. They sum it up by saying, "Retinoids are the only thing you can put on your skin that can repair sun damage, giving you less wrinkled skin."

At the conclusion of a recent study at the University of Michigan, researchers found that use of creams containing retinol actually reversed skin aging. In addition, they discovered that vitamin A, the main component in retinol creams, has been shown to speed up the rate at which the body sheds dead skin, while stimulating collagen production, which makes the skin look plumper and fine lines look smoother.

It's no wonder retinol remains a staple in many skincare preparations today. I like to refer to it as the Fountain of Youth.

Spin Trap

Also known as phenyl-butyl-nitrone (PBN), spin trap is one of the latest advances in antiaging technology in skincare today. Spin trap is a form of nitrogen and functions as an antioxidant, but not in the traditional way.

Rather than simply destroying free radicals, it restores balance to unstable molecules. Spin trap converts the rogue free radicals back into vital oxygen and redirects them for the deepest tissue respiration, which is necessary for all healthy cells. Scientists have proven that nitrone spin trap is highly effective in reversing the signs of aging in the skin. It literally defends the skin against free radicals and other environmental damage, hence earning its name – the intelligent antioxidant.

In his book *The Wrinkle Cure*, Dr. Perricone notes that spin traps are capable of "stopping free-radical damage before it begins," and notes that these agents "create a barrier – a trap – that holds free radicals in place" so that they can be "stopped before they scar the cells that make up your skin." Dr. Perricone also explains that researchers found that the traps "actually prevented the free radicals from moving from place to place and damaging cells."

It's easy to see why spin traps have found their way into many skincare preparations, including creams, serums and masks. For years I have included spin traps in many of my skincare products because they are amazingly effective in protecting the skin from myriad sources of damage.

Newest Advances in Skincare

Plant Stem Cells

Stem cells are the most important cells in the skin. In fact, they are the source for continuous regeneration of the epidermis, as well as the formation of new hair and hair pigments. Reduced viability and premature apoptosis (death) of stem cells is a principal cause of tissue aging. Studies have found that using cultured stem-cell extracts from Uttwiler Spätlauber apples in skincare preparations has been enormously effective in the fight against aging. The reason is, perhaps, that these particular apples stay fresh for an extraordinary length of time, and it appears that their stem-cell extracts have a special epigenetic profile that resists cell apoptosis (cell death), promotes regeneration of skin and hair, and delays the appearance of skin aging.

Fiflow

Oxygen is essential to the skin. Pollution and other environmental problems have effectively lowered the overall oxygen level of the air to about half of what it used to be. The result is that oxygen depletion and carbon dioxide accumulation are causing poor cell respiration, leading to dehydration, uneven skin tone and dull skin. Poor air quality is probably the largest contributor to the premature aging of the skin, as carbon dioxide hinders or actually stops bio-pathways for cell metabolism.

PFCs (perfluorocarbons) are the best gas carriers known to science and are entirely drug free. Fiflow BTX is based on a blend of medical-grade PFCs, and studies show that its use results in increased skin moisture and volume, and long-term improvement of age lines.

Longevicell

Longevicell, obtained from myrtle, a Mediterranean shrub, is rich in oligo-galacturonans and prized for its rejuvenating properties. Longevicell is said to act by regulating the process involved in skin longevity, regulating the proteins involved in cell-to-cell communication and helping to prevent your collagen from becoming stiff. Studies have shown that Longevicell can effectively slow down the aging process in the skin, promote cell longevity and regenerate skin tissue cells.

Venuceane

Environmental factors, such as overexposure to the sun's UVA rays, contribute to premature aging of the skin. Venuceane is derived from a culture of the *Thermus thermophillus* organism, which lives in the Guaymas basin in the Gulf of California. It is known for its strong antioxidant properties and free-radical protection. It has increasing efficacy with rising temperatures and is stable when it is in contact with UV rays. It has been shown to adapt and maintain the skin's natural protection enzymes, reducing DNA damage caused by UVA irradiation and even repairing sun-damaged skin.

Kombucha

Derived from fermented sweet black tea, kombucha, also known as a "long-life fungus," is rich in organic acids and B vitamins. Tests have shown it to inhibit a reaction in the skin that can lead to stiffening of the skin cells and collagen, decrease skin roughness, and create a re-densifying effect by increasing the adipocyte population from fibroblast activity. Hence, the name kombucha has become synonymous with the term "lipofilling effect." It is said to increase the overall skin quality by enhancing smoothness, radiance and color.

Mitoprotect

All our cells need energy to maintain their health, including skin cells. Mitroprotect was formulated as a form of skin nutrition to enhance, support and protect the mitochondria, which is the part of the cell known as the "powerhouse." Mitoprotect combines five key ingredients – the skincare wonders spin trap (PBN), coenzyme Q10, R-lipoic acid, adenine and acetyl-L carnitine – to nourish, protect against free-radical damage, support the function of the mitochondria in our skin cells, aid the regeneration of the cells and remodel the collagen production in our skin. Studies have shown that Mitoprotect can help keep the skin looking young and more energetic.

All these products and fantastic new skincare ingredients have a role to play in creating and maintaining healthy, younger-looking skin. Alongside a healthy diet, good, restful sleep (on your back!) and dry-brushing, they can help to ensure that you give your skin the very best chance of defying the effects of aging. However, there is no doubt that the structure on which your skin sits – the muscles that make it move, and help provide the definition of your face – must be worked, too. And that's where Ultimate Facercise comes in!

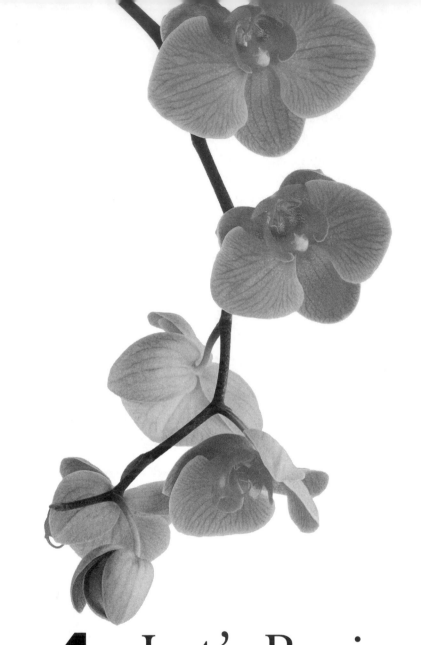

4 Let's Begin – The Ultimate Facercise Program!

Before we start, bear in mind that if you have never exercised your face before, you cannot make up for lost time by overdoing it. By overdoing it, I mean performing the exercises more than the prescribed number of sets a day which, in this case, would be two sets a day.

Overworking the muscles of the face can often have the reverse effect. When the muscles of the face are worked to the point of fatigue, you need to allow them proper time to rest and recuperate – and then to grow. If you are feeling impatient, remember that you cannot make up for years of neglect by doing more than the prescribed number of sets a day. Anything worth doing is worth doing well, and at the right pace.

I've had clients call me in a panic to say that everything was going fine – their face was looking good, they were seeing improvements – and now, all of a sudden, it is sagging again. I usually go through what they are doing to get to the bottom of it. Invariably, it emerges that they are trying to create the face of their dreams in just a few short days. It doesn't work like that. You simply cannot perform the exercises four, five or six times a day and not expect to see your face regress. Muscles that are overworked like that have basically been stripped. They have not been allowed to rest, recuperate and build. Trust me, you will not need to suffer through any awkward periods with Facercise, as I have spent many, many years honing, tweaking and perfecting the Facercise technique. You just need to be consistent and patient, and stick to the plan. Exercise your face by performing the entire program twice daily and then call it a day.

13 Essential Exercises

These 13 exercises form the backbone of the Ultimate Facercise program and should be undertaken as suggested to create youthful, tighter, healthier skin on your face. Before we start, however, there are a few things that will help make the program work at optimal level.

Secrets of Facercise Success

Posture

As you prepare to perform each exercise, pull your navel back toward your spine, as far as you can. Wrap (tighten) your thighs and buttocks. Your nipples are now called headlights and you want them on high beam. Push your face forward and your shoulders back for resistance. Hold this position while you do the exercises. This posture acts as an anchor and allows you to focus on the individual facial muscles you are exercising. Many of my clients have told me that a very pleasant side effect of this posturing position is that their hips actually become smaller. I would say that's quite a nice side effect! Going forward, whenever you see the words "Assume the basic posture," this is the position to which I am referring. This posturing technique will enhance the effect of the exercises.

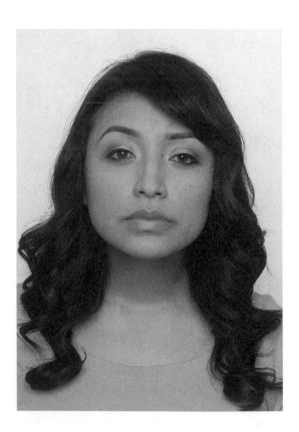 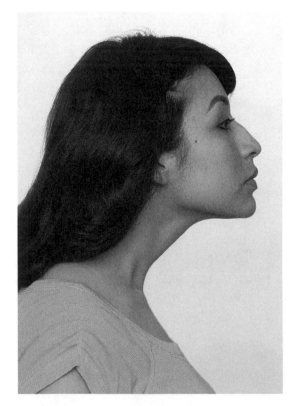

Lactic-Acid Burn

Concentrate on the muscle group you are working until you feel that tight, achy, burning sensation. The exertion creates a lactic-acid buildup in the muscle and the burning sensation is a sign that the muscle is being worked to its maximum capacity. While performing certain exercises like the Lip Plumper (see page 72), you may not feel a burning, but rather a tingling numbness or a thickening sensation. During the Furrow Smoother exercise (see page 63), you may feel more of a tightening sensation. These sensations are all still considered "getting the burn."

Using your fingertips on your face as counterweights while performing facial exercises creates resistance and works the muscles harder. As a result, the muscles will grow stronger and you will achieve results more quickly.

You'll come across the term "pulsing," which means moving your fingers quickly up and down on the muscle to intensify the feeling of the lactic-acid burn. Don't forget this, as I use this instruction in every exercise – and believe me, it works!

Visualization

Visualize and feel the energy moving through your muscles as they work. In your mind, imagine your muscles starting to lift and move up your face. Whenever I use the term "energy," I am referring to the concept of energy flow. Energy flow is based on the Chinese medicinal theory that energy moves in pathways around the body. I know from experience that when clients can actually feel and visualize energy flow, they learn the exercise techniques even quicker. Also, utilizing the visualization technique creates even more rapid muscle growth than you would experience without using your imagination.

Ache Away

To relax your facial muscles after performing each exercise, press your lips together and blow out between them, feeling a vibrating sensation. It's the same sound you'd make if you blew bubbles with your lips in the bathtub. We all remember doing that as kids. You will be doing this after each exercise to relax your face and "blow away" that achy feeling.

Exercise 1
The Eye Opener

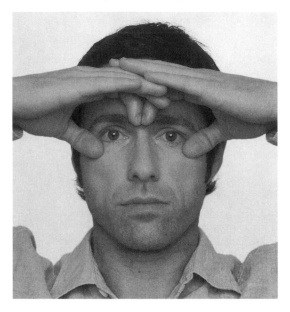
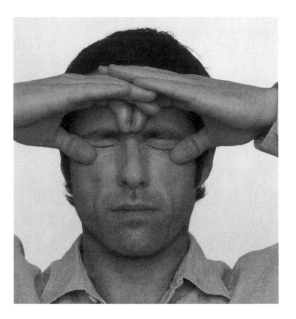

Technique

You can perform this exercise lying down or in a sitting position. Assume the basic posture (see page 60). Place your two index fingers together between your brows. Wrap your thumbs lightly around the outer-eye corners, as if you have a pair of sunglasses around your eyes.

Squeeze your eyes shut tightly – as tight as you are squeezing your buttocks – pull your two index fingers up slightly between your brows and pull your thumbs up toward the top of your ears. Re-squeeze your eyes shut very tight. Breathe normally. Push your face forward and shoulders back for added resistance.

Hold and count to 40.

Benefits

The Eye Opener exercises the *orbicularis oculi* muscle, which surrounds the entire eye. This muscle opens and closes the eye. It also tones the upper and lower eyelids and reduces under-eye puffiness, making your eyes appear larger, younger and more alert.

Tip

Perform the Eye Opener twice a day. If you have deep hollows or severe under-eye puffiness, repeat three times daily. Clients have remarked that this exercise also reduces sinus headaches.

Use slight pressure with your index fingers between the brows. Pull index fingers up slightly but don't lift fingers off your face. Keep your thumbs at your outer-eye corners, using light pressure, and pull your thumbs up toward your ears – don't lift them off your face.

Exercise 2
• •
The Furrow Smoother

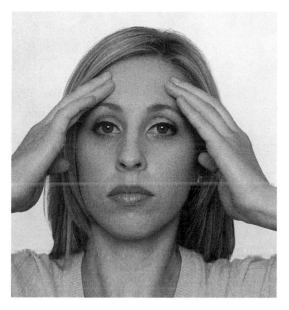
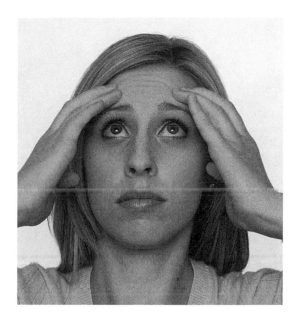

Technique

You can do this exercise in a sitting position or lying down. Assume the basic posture. Spread your fingers across the center of your forehead. Pull your fingertips down against your brows. Push your eyebrows up and hold that tension. Look up to the ceiling. Push your face forward and your shoulders back for resistance. Keep your eyebrows pushed up and fingers pulling down. Push your feet into the floor for added resistance. Keep going until you feel a burn or a tension in your forehead.

Hold for a count of 30.

Benefits

This exercise works the *epicranius*, which raises the eyebrows; the *frontalis*, which draws the scalp forward; the *occipitalis*, which draws the scalp back; and the *galea aponeurotica*, which joins the *frontalis* and the *occipitalis*. It also raises the eyebrows and diminishes hooding of the upper eyelids, as well as getting rid of those question-mark lines between the brows and the lines on the forehead.

Tip

Do the Furrow Smoother twice daily. To correct heavy question-mark lines, repeat this exercise three times a day. If your fingers slip, use a piece of tissue on your forehead underneath your fingers for better traction. I also suggest sleeping at night with surgical tape over the question-mark or forehead lines. This allows the muscles to relax while dreaming and you will quickly see softened lines when you waken.

Exercise 3
The Lower Eyelid Lifter

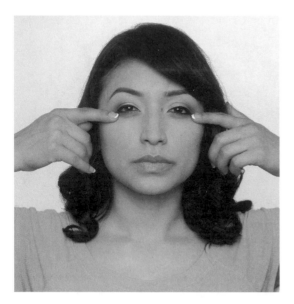
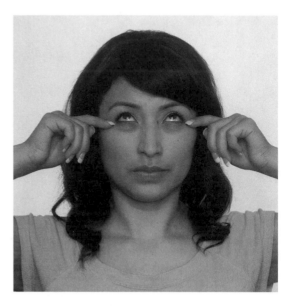

Technique

You can do this exercise sitting up or lying down. Assume the basic posture. Place your index fingers lightly at your outer-eye corners. Place them where you can feel the lower eyelashes. Make a strong squint up with your lower eyelids. You should feel the outer-eye muscles pulse. Look up to the ceiling. Push your face forward and your shoulders back for resistance. Push your feet into the floor for added resistance.

Hold the squint for a count of 40.

Benefits

This exercise strengthens the *orbicularis oculi* muscle, firming the lower eyelid, diminishing under-eye hollows and reducing under-eye puffiness.

Tip

Perform the Lower Eyelid Lifter twice a day. If you have excessive under-eye puffiness, repeat this exercise three times a day.

Exercise 4
The Face Filler

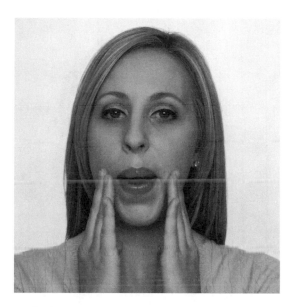

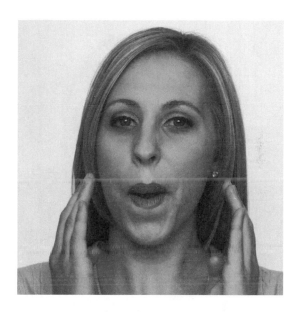

Technique

This exercise works best in a sitting position. Assume the basic posture. Open your mouth and wrap the corners of your mouth inside, pulling them toward your back teeth. Keep your upper lip pressing down against your teeth. Keep your lower lip snug against your teeth.

Draw an imaginary line with your fingers from your mouth corners to your back teeth, to keep your point of focus. Make a small mouth, not like a smile. Push your face forward and your shoulders back. Push your feet against the floor for added resistance.

Place your fingers on your face at your wrapped-in mouth corners. Make small circular motions on your face to help widen and expand your face. Keep your mouth corners pulling in tight toward your back teeth.

Start to pull your fingers away from your mouth corners, continuing to make small circles as you feel your face widen. Push your feet against the floor for added resistance. Continue until you feel the burn on the side of your face and make 30 quick circles with your fingers to intensify the burn.

Blow out between your lips.

Benefit

This exercise can help create symmetry as well as widen and soften a thin, gaunt face.

Tip

Do this exercise two to three times a day, depending on how thin your face is. Avoid this exercise if your face is already wide.

Exercise 5
The Cheek Energizer

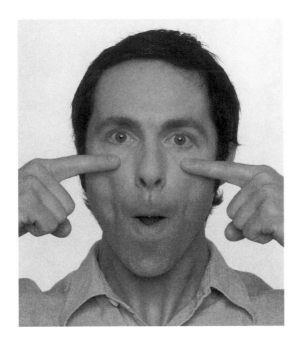 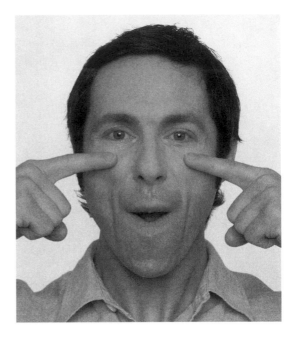

Technique

This exercise can be performed while sitting up or lying down. Make a long, narrow "O" with your mouth, pulling your upper and lower lips away from each other as firmly as you can. Keep your upper lip pressing down against your teeth.

Place both of your hands on the outside of your face and then move them into the middle of your face to bring the energy field into the center of your face. Place your index fingers lightly on top of your cheeks.

Smile with the middle of your upper lip, while thinking the expression "Eww" (the sound you might make if you just smelled something disgusting). Keep your upper and lower lips firmly pulling away from each other. Feel your cheeks move under your index fingers.

Repeat the smile and release, thinking the expression "Eww" 20 times.

Stop thinking "Eww" and keep your long "O" very strong. Push your face forward and your shoulders back for resistance. Look up to the ceiling. Move your index fingers up to the top of your head as you smile with your upper lip pushing the energy up under your cheeks. If sitting up, push your feet against the floor to move the energy up stronger.

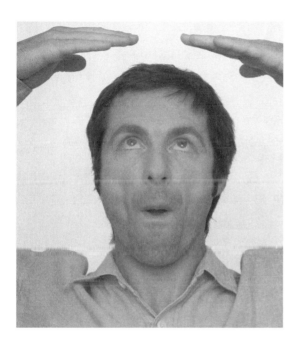

Pulse your hands above your head and count to 30.

Benefits

The Cheek Energizer exercises the *buccinator* muscle. This muscle forms the rounded top part of the cheek. You are also working the *orbicularis oris*, which is the circular muscle surrounding the mouth. It enlarges the cheeks and fills in the hollows under the eyes. The *quadratus labii superioris* is working to counteract the lengthening and flattening effects of gravity. The Cheek Energizer removes the tired, stressed look that the face develops during the course of a busy day, and increases blood circulation, giving your complexion a rosy, youthful glow.

Tip

Do the Cheek Energizer twice a day. If you are under unusual stress, do this exercise as often as necessary. Keep the energy in the middle of your face, so that you don't engage your jaw hinge. Open your mouth by pulling your lips apart, not by using your jaw hinge.

Exercise 6
The Nose Transformer

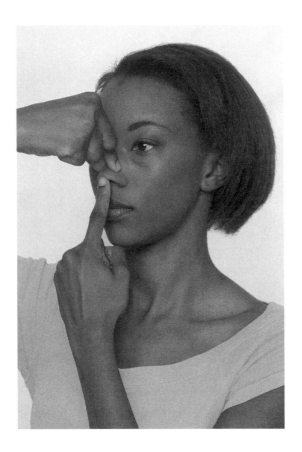

Repeat the exercise 40 times. You should feel the nose tip push against your finger each time. Breathe at a normal rate while you perform these repetitions.

Benefits

The Nose Transformer exercises the *depressor septi* muscle, which shortens and narrows the nose tip. The nose continues to widen and grow throughout our lives, and this helps it retain a youthful, firmer shape.

Exercising our nose stimulates blood circulation and oxygen flow throughout the entire upper lip and nose area. You will feel a tingling sensation around the nose, which is a sign of increased blood circulation. A well-toned nose can even hide imperfections like a nose bump.

Tip

Do the Nose Transformer exercise once a day for general toning, and twice a day if your nose is too wide or too long. Clients who have had rhinoplasty surgery reported that doing this exercise for several weeks helped to give their nose a more naturally sculpted look and they healed more quickly.

Technique

You can do this exercise sitting up or lying down. Grasp the bridge of your nose with your thumb and index finger. Pinch the bridge and push your thumb and index finger toward your face. Push your nose tip up firmly with your other index finger. Flex your nose down by pulling your upper lip down over your teeth or by pushing your nostrils down. Hold for a second then release the lip.

Alternative Version of the Nose Transformer

This technique helps straighten a crooked nose. Many of my clients who were contemplating rhinoplasty surgery were thrilled that they were able to avoid it by straightening their noses with this technique.

Technique

You can do this exercise sitting up or lying down. Grasp the bridge of your nose with your thumb and index finger. Pinch the bridge and push your thumb and index finger toward your face. Push your nose tip up firmly *in the opposite direction of the crook* with your index finger. Flex your nose down by pulling your upper lip down over your teeth or by pushing your nostrils down. Hold for a second then release the lip.

Repeat the exercise 40 times. You should feel the nose tip push against your finger each time. Breathe at a normal rate while you perform these repetitions.

Tip

Perform this exercise twice daily to straighten a crooked nose. Clients who have followed this technique have been able to straighten their noses effectively in a very short period of time.

Continue to push your nose tip up *firmly in the opposite direction of the crook* even after you have straightened it to maintain the straightened effect.

Exercise 7
The Lip Lift

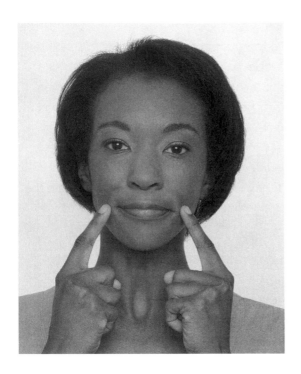

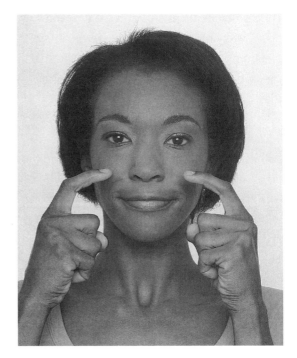

Technique

This exercise is most effective when sitting in an upright position. Press your lips together, but do not purse them. Tighten the corners of your mouth into balls. Do not make a smile with your mouth. Squeeze the corners of your mouth as though you were sucking on two small lemons. Do not clench your teeth. Push your face forward and your shoulders back for resistance.

Tap your index fingers at the corners of your mouth. Keep squeezing your mouth corners as you visualize the corners of your mouth turning up into a tiny smile. Now visualize the corners turning down, resembling a tiny frown. Move your fingers away from the corners of your mouth and make tiny up-and-down motions with your fingers to follow the visualization of your mouth corners moving up and down.

Continue moving your fingers in small

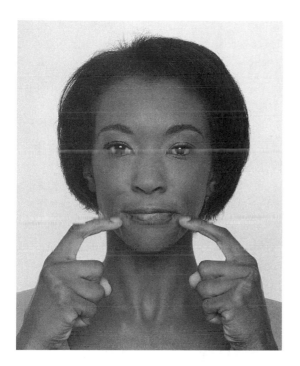

Benefits

As we age, the *zygomaticus* muscles sag, causing the mouth corners to droop. The Lip Lift will firm the mouth corners, turning them up into a more youthful position. Many women say they started exercising their faces when their mouths started to look like their mother's.

Tip

This is a visualization exercise. You are *mentally* moving your mouth corners up and down, not *physically* moving them. Perform this exercise twice daily to keep mother's mouth away.

up-and-down motions until you experience a burning sensation in the mouth corners.

Pulse your index fingers up and down quickly for a count of 40 to intensify the burn. You are feeling the lactic-acid burn, which means you are working the muscle to its maximum capacity.

To release the lactic-acid burn, press your lips together and blow between them, making sure that you vibrate your lips.

Exercise 8
The Lip Plumper

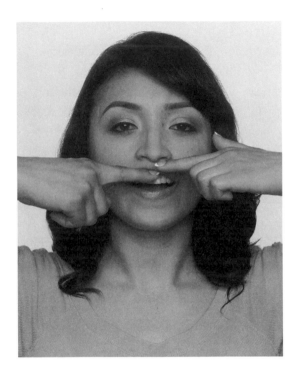

Technique

This exercise can be done either lying down or sitting up. Curl your upper lip under itself, pressing up against your upper teeth gumline. Hold it up with your index finger (if necessary). Tap the center of your upper lip with your other index finger. Visualize that you are crushing a ball in the center of your lip.

Tap the center of your lip with your index finger and slowly pull your finger away from your lip in small circular motions to mimic the ball shape. When you start to feel a burn – or numbness or a thickening of your lip – make 20 quick circular motions with your finger.

Now visualize that you are crushing a ball at each mouth corner. With one hand, tap your thumb at one corner and your index finger at the other corner of your mouth. Keep your upper lip curled under and pressing up against your upper teeth gumline, while holding it up with your index finger (if necessary). Repeat the exercise.

Go until you feel a burn or numbness in your mouth corners and then make 20 quick circular motions with your thumb and index finger.

Release the lactic acid by blowing out through your pressed lips.

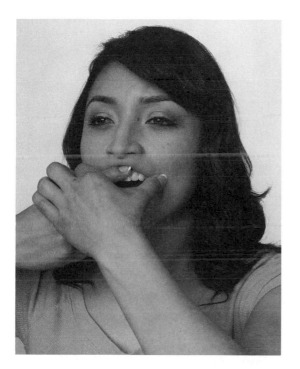

Benefits

Exercising the *orbicularis oris* muscle around the mouth makes the mouth look fuller, younger and firmer without the expense of costly fillers. This exercise enlarges the lips, restores their rosy pink color and smoothes out the liplines.

Tip

Do the Lip Plumper twice a day to plump up thin lips. Repeat the Lip Plumper exercise four times a day for that "red carpet" Angelina Jolie look. My personal tip is to perform this exercise four times a day and line your lips twice with lipliner, staying on the border of the lip, and filling in with a glossy lipstick. You will definitely have that celebrity look.

Exercise 9
• •
The Nasolabial Plumper

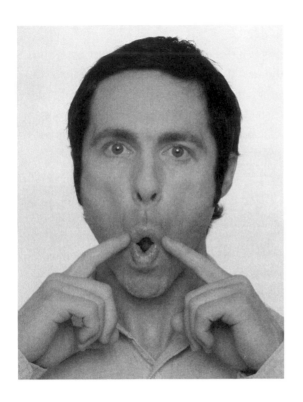
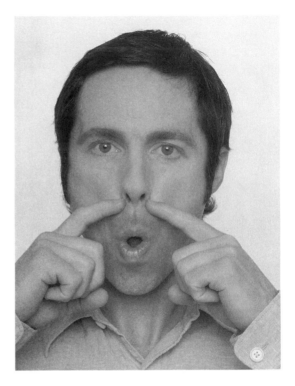

Technique

This exercise is most effective when sitting in an upright position. Assume the basic posture. Make a long, narrow "O" with your mouth. Think an oval shape. Keep your upper lip pressing down against your teeth. Place your hands on the outside of your face and move them into the middle to bring the energy field into the center of your face. Push your face forward and your shoulders back. Push your feet into the floor for added resistance.

Place your index fingers at your mouth corners. Slowly move your index fingers up the nasolabial line from your mouth corners to your nose corners, going *very slowly*, as if you were moving the energy through mud. When your fingers are at the nose corners, *very slowly* move your fingers

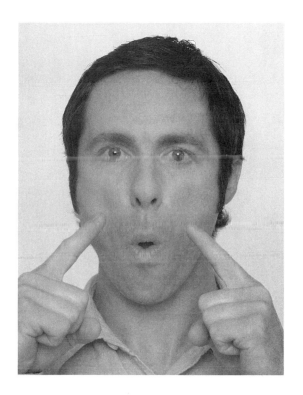

Benefits

By exercising the *dilator naris anterior* and the *dilator naris posterior* muscles, you will plump out and smooth the line formed from the nose corners to the mouth corners.

Tip

As you visualize the energy from the mouth corners to the nose corners, you need to go *very slowly,* moving the imaginary energy from the mouth corners to the nose corners, and the nose corners to the mouth corners. The slower you go, the faster you will create the burn. Keep your mouth in a *firm* long "O" position. Sleeping on your face further compresses and deepens this line, so sleep on your back to avoid exaggerating this line.

down toward the mouth corners, again as if you were moving the energy through mud. Keep repeating this movement up and down, until you feel the burn in the nasolabial line.

Pulse your fingers up and down quickly for a count of 30.

Now blow out between your lips.

Exercise 10
The Neck Toner

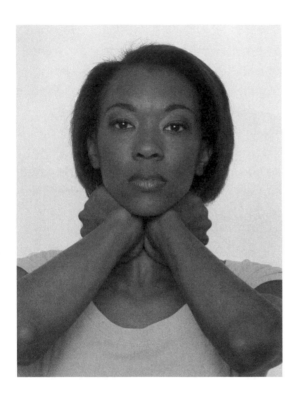

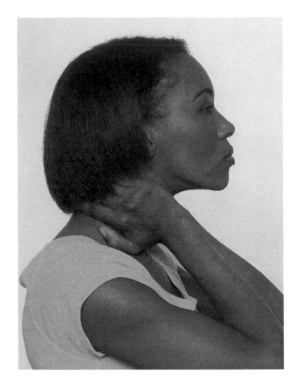

Technique

This exercise offers two different positions, which can be adopted according to your physical capability. If you have a healthy back and neck, you can do both positions. If not, only perform the exercise in position 1.

Position 1 – Sitting Up

Grasp the front of your neck with the palms of your hands as if you were choking yourself. Make sure your palms are touching your neck.

Assume the basic posture. Push your head out away from your body with the front of your neck and release. Repeat 20 times.

Position 2 – Lying Down

With your legs bent and feet on the floor, place your hands down by your sides. Suck your belly button into your spine, tighten your buttocks and lift your head straight up off the floor an inch or so, lifting and leading

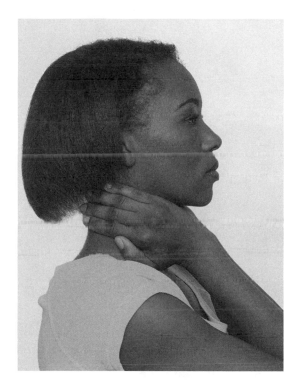

Benefits

This exercise works the *platysma*, the *sterno-cleidomastoid* and the *trapezius* muscles of the neck. These muscles allow us to hold our heads upright. Strengthening your neck will smooth and firm sagging neck skin. Clients have said their necks have become so strong that it has helped avert whiplash from car accidents. No more hiding your neck behind turtlenecks and scarves!

Tip

Do the Neck Toner twice daily. Be sure to lift your head with the front of your neck and tightened buttocks, *not the back of your neck and head*. Remember the expression "pain in the neck"? You want to avoid that!

with the front of your neck and tightened buttocks.

Do not lift with the back of your neck or head. Turn your head from side to side 20 times, then relax.

Build up to 30 times.

Exercise 11
The Jaw Toner

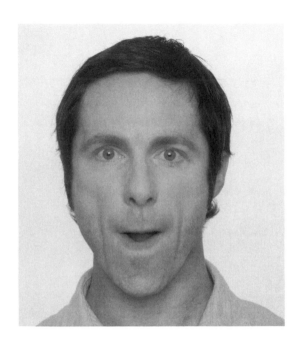

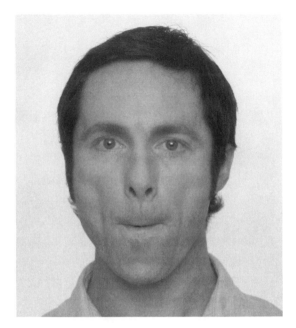

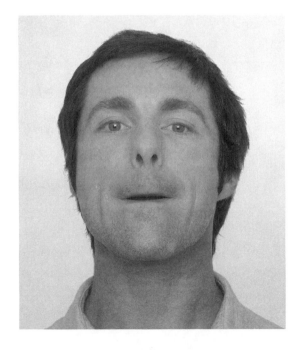

Technique

Perform this exercise while sitting up. Assume the basic posture. Open your mouth and roll your lower lip in over your bottom teeth. Wrap the corners of your mouth inside, pulling them toward your back teeth. Make a small mouth, not like a smile. Keep your upper lip pressing down against your teeth. Push your feet against the floor for added resistance.

Slowly open and close your mouth five times, as if your mouth corners and chin were connected, working together to close your mouth. *Hold*. Pull your chin up toward the ceiling about an inch. Open and close your mouth slowly five times. *Hold*. Pull your chin up toward the ceiling another inch. *Hold*.

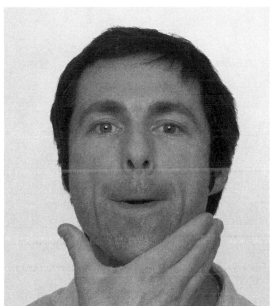

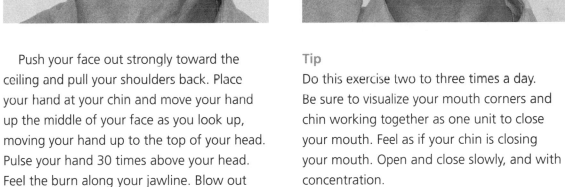

Push your face out strongly toward the ceiling and pull your shoulders back. Place your hand at your chin and move your hand up the middle of your face as you look up, moving your hand up to the top of your head. Pulse your hand 30 times above your head. Feel the burn along your jawline. Blow out between your lips.

Benefits

The Jaw Toner benefits the *pterygold internus* muscle in the jaw. This exercise will give you a well-defined, toned jawline. Many clients and dentists have agreed that this exercise relieves painful symptoms of TMJ (temporo-mandibular joint syndrome).

Tip

Do this exercise two to three times a day. Be sure to visualize your mouth corners and chin working together as one unit to close your mouth. Feel as if your chin is closing your mouth. Open and close slowly, and with concentration.

Exercise 12
The Face Contour

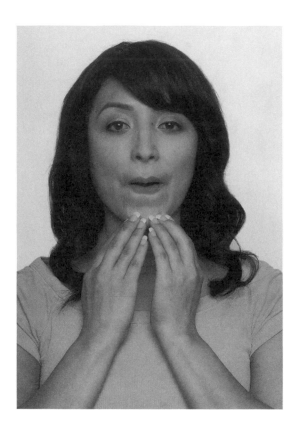

Technique

Do this exercise sitting up. Assume the basic posture. Open your mouth and roll your lips over your teeth. Pull the corners of your mouth in toward your back teeth. Keep your mouth small, not like a smile. Draw an imaginary line with your fingers from your mouth corners to your back teeth to keep your point of focus on your back teeth. Keep your mouth corners tightly wrapped in toward your back teeth. Place your fingers on your chin. Push your face forward and shoulders back.

Slowly move your fingers up along the sides of your face as you visualize the sides of your face lifting. Look up to the ceiling. Push your feet against the floor for resistance. Continue moving your fingers up along the sides of your face to the tops of your ears. *Hold*.

Pulse your hands above your ears for a count of 40. Feel the burn along the sides of your face.

Blow out between your lips.

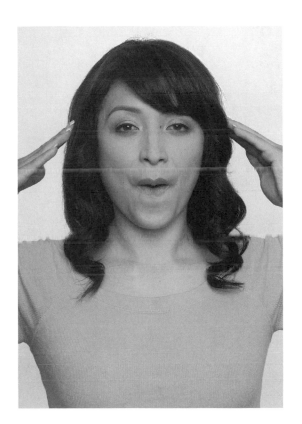

Benefits

The Face Contour will narrow a too wide face. If your face is thin, it will keep the sides of your face toned and lifted. Exercising the *buccinator* muscle will increase overall facial tone.

Tip

If your face is wide or full, do this exercise twice daily. If your face is thin, perform the Face Contour exercise once a day for overall toning

Exercise 13
The Neck and Chin Lift

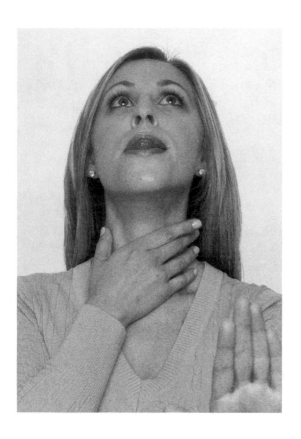

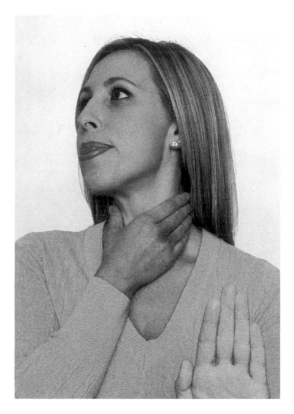

Technique

Sit tall and straight with your belly sucked into your spine. Tighten your buttocks and put your headlights on high beam. Place one hand on the front of your neck with light pressure, and one hand on the wall or work surface. Point your chin up to the ceiling. Smile strongly, pushing out your tongue and curling it up toward your nose. Look up to the ceiling.

Push away from the wall with your hand quickly, as if you were a rocking chair. Push away from the wall each time like a rocking chair, rocking backward, not forward, toward the wall. Rock 30 times.

Turn your head to the right and look over your shoulder. Rock 30 times. Turn your head to the left and look over your shoulder. Rock 30 times.

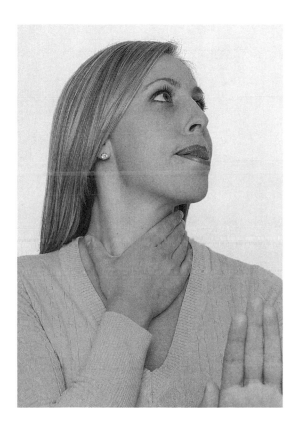

Tip

Do this exercise twice daily. Be sure to hold your chin up high, without causing pain.

Benefits

The Neck and Chin Lift exercise strengthens the *platysma* muscle and firms the chin, neck and jawline.

Double chins – *be gone!*

5

Ultimate Facercise in the Car — A Short Program

I know many of you lead busy lives and I want you to achieve your personal goals with the Ultimate Facercise program. So I've modified the exercises to allow you to do them in the car while driving to work or school or running your daily errands.

The only exercise you must do at a red light or while the car is not in motion is the Eye Opener (see page 62). Remember to be careful and watch for traffic lights and, of course, other vehicles.

Remember: Do not endanger yourself or others. Take care while you Facercise in the car, even at very slow speeds.

Car Exercise 1: The Eye Opener
CAUTION: Do this exercise only when stopped at a traffic light or stop sign.

Place your index fingers together between your brows with light pressure. Wrap your thumbs around the outer-eye corners, as if you have a pair of sunglasses around your eyes. Squeeze your eyes shut tight. Count to 40. Every few counts, peek with one eye to see if your traffic light has changed, and continue to squeeze eyes shut tightly. Count to 30.

Car Exercise 2: The Furrow Smoother
Spread the fingers of one hand out across the middle of your forehead. Pull your fingers down so that they are above the brows. Push your eyebrows up hard. You will feel a strong band of pressure across your forehead. Hold and count to 20 while pushing away from the steering wheel. This will intensify the energy.

Car Exercise 3: The Lower Eyelid Lifter
Place your right thumb at the outer-eye corner of your right eye and your right index finger at the outer corner of your left eye. Squint up hard with your lower eyelid. Push away from the steering wheel for a count of 40. Keep your eyes wide open *and on the road ahead.*

Car Exercise 4:   The Face Filler

Open your mouth and pull the corners of your mouth inside toward the back teeth and roll them in tightly. Keep your upper lip firmly pressed down against the teeth. Keep your lower lip pressing against the teeth. Make a small mouth, not like a smile.

Place the thumb and index finger of one hand on your face at the corners of your mouth. Make small circular motions on your face as you visualize big fat cheeks coming out of the corners of your mouth. Continue making small circular motions until you begin to feel the muscle widen.

Slowly pull your fingers away from your face, while continuing to make circular motions, and push against the steering wheel for added resistance. When you begin to feel the lactic-acid burn in the sides of your face, make rapid circles with your fingers to intensify and enhance the burn. Count to 30.

Car Exercise 5:   The Cheek Energizer

Open your mouth and pull the upper and lower lips away from each other to form a long, strong, narrow oval shape. Keep the long oval shape of the mouth. Press the upper lip firmly against the teeth. Place the thumb and index finger of one hand on top of your cheeks. Smile with the middle of your upper lip, thinking the expression "Eww" (the sound you might make if you just smelled something disgusting). Push the muscle up under the cheek each time you smile. You will feel the cheek muscles move under your fingers. Repeat this movement 20 times.

You can push away from the steering wheel each time you smile and release, to intensify the energy.

On the twentieth smile, forcefully pull the upper and lower lips away from each other. Slowly move your thumb and index fingers off your cheeks and up to the roof of the car as you visualize moving the energy from the middle of your face to above your head. Pulse your hand above your head and count to 20.

Car Exercise 6:   The Nose Transformer

Use your index finger to push the tip of your nose up and hold it firmly in place. Flex your nose down by pulling your upper lip down over your teeth. Hold for a second before releasing your lip. Repeat this movement 30 times. You will feel the nose tip push against the finger each time.

If you have a crooked nose, push your nose tip up firmly in the opposite direction of the crook. Repeat the technique.

Car Exercise 7: The Lip Lift

Press your lips together. *Do not* purse them. Tighten the corners of your mouth into hard knots. Don't make a smile. Squeeze the corners only, as if sucking on a lemon at each corner. Do not clench your teeth.

Tap your thumb and index finger at the corners of your mouth. Pull them away from the corners in small up-and-down movements as you visualize the mouth corners turning up an inch and then down an inch. Continue this movement until you feel a lactic-acid burn.

Hold for a count of 30, pushing away from the steering wheel, and pulse your thumb and index finger up and down to intensify the burn.

Car Exercise 8: The Lip Plumper

Curl your upper lip in and press it against your upper teeth gumline. Visualize crushing a ball in the middle of your lip. Tap the center of your lip with your index finger. Pull your finger away slowly in a circular motion to mimic the ball shape, until you feel a lactic-acid burn.

Make quick circles with your finger to a count of 15. Tap the corners of your mouth with your thumb and index finger where you are visualizing two more balls.

Repeat the exercise, pushing against the steering wheel for increased energy. Keep the upper lip curled in and pressing up against the gumline for the entire exercise. Go for the burn and make 20 quick circles with your thumb and index finger.

Car Exercise 9: The Nasolabial Plumper

Open your mouth and pull the upper and lower lips away from each other, forming a long, narrow oval shape. Keep the long, narrow oval shape of the mouth. Keep your upper lip pressed firmly against the teeth. Visualize a line of energy moving very, very slowly from your mouth corners up to the sides of your nostrils. Use the thumb and index finger of one hand to track this line of energy upward. Feel as if you are pushing the energy through mud. Push against the steering wheel as you slowly move the energy up and down the nasolabial line.

Next, visualize the line of energy moving back down that imaginary line toward your mouth corners. Go very, very slowly, as if you are moving the energy through mud. Keep repeating this energy movement very slowly up and down, using your thumb and index finger to follow and intensify the energy. Continue until you feel the burn.

Push against the steering wheel and then pulse your fingers up and down for a count of 20.

Car Exercise 10:   The Neck Toner

Grasp the front of your neck with one hand, as if you were choking yourself. Push your chin away from your body with the front of your neck and toward the windshield, then relax. Push away from the steering wheel each time you push your chin away from your body.

Repeat this action 20 times. You should feel the muscles in front of your neck flex each time.

Car Exercise 11:   The Jaw Toner

Open your mouth and roll your lower lip in tightly over the lower teeth. Pull the corners of your mouth inside toward the back teeth and roll them in tightly. Keep your upper lip pressing down firmly against the teeth. Make a small mouth, not like a smile.

Open and close your mouth five times slowly, as if your mouth corners and chin are connected, working together to close your mouth. Hold.

Tilt your chin up about an inch. Open and close your mouth five times slowly. Hold.

Tilt your chin up about an inch. Push against the steering wheel for resistance. Feel the burn along your jawline and hold for a count of 30.

Car Exercise 12:   The Face Contour

Open your mouth and roll your lips over your teeth. Pull the corners of your mouth inside toward the back teeth, and roll them in tightly. Keep your mouth small, not like a smile. Place your hand at your chin. Slowly move your hand up the middle of your face as you visualize the sides of your face moving up past the jawline and the top of your head. Push away from the steering wheel for increased resistance.

Continue visualizing the energy moving up along the sides of your face until you feel the burn. Then pulse your hand above your head for a count of 30.

Car Exercise 13:   The Neck and Chin Lift

Place one hand on the front of your neck. Grasp your neck, as if you are choking yourself. Sit up straight, pulling your belly button to your spine, and tighten your buttocks. Pull your back slightly away from the seat. Hold your chin up high, but not so high that you disrupt your line of vision. Stick out your tongue, pointing it toward your nose, and smile. Push away from the steering wheel as if you were a rocking chair. You will be pushing the energy back like a rocking chair, *not* rocking forward toward the steering wheel. Rock 35 times.

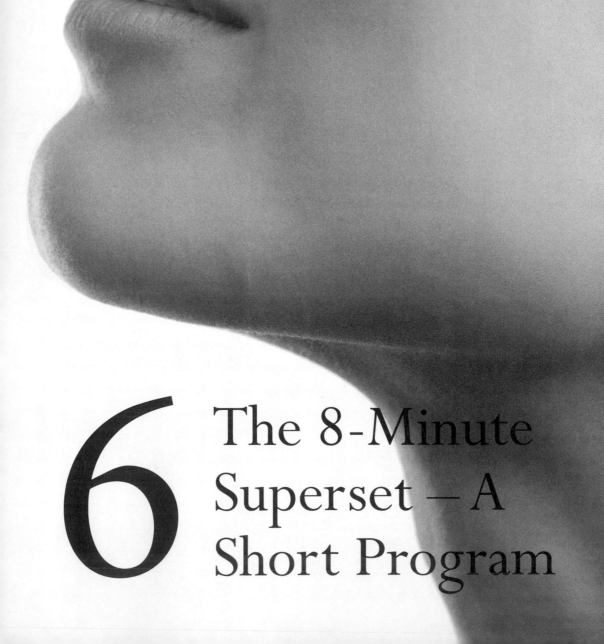

6

The 8-Minute Superset — A Short Program

Use this technique only after you have learned the exercises from the detailed instructions. These exercises should be used when you have limited time, but don't dare miss performing your daily Ultimate Facercise routine.

Exercise 1: The Eye Opener

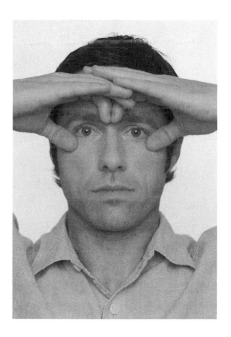 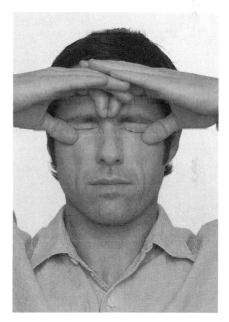

Place index fingers between the brows. Wrap thumbs around your outer-eye corners. Squeeze eyes shut tight. Face forward, shoulders back. Push your feet against the floor for resistance.

Hold and count to 30.

Exercise 2: The Furrow Smoother

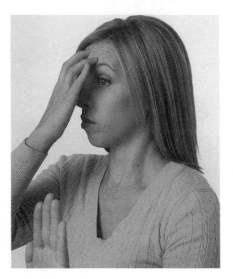 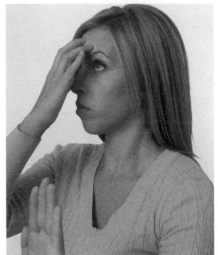

Place one hand on wall or work surface, pushing away for resistance. Spread fingers across brow. Pull fingers down toward brows and push up brows. Face forward, shoulders back. Push your feet against the floor for resistance.

Hold and count to 20.

Exercise 3: The Lower Eyelid Lifter

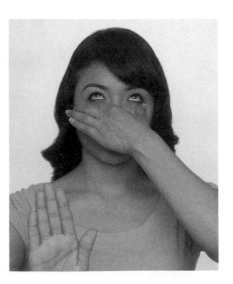

Place one hand on wall or work surface, pushing away for resistance. Place your thumb and index finger at your outer-eye corners. Squint up strong. Face forward, shoulders back. Push your feet against the floor for resistance.

Hold for a count of 30.

Exercise 4: The Face Filler

Place one hand on wall or work surface, pushing away for resistance. Open your mouth and pull mouth corners inside toward back teeth. Push face forward, shoulders back. Place thumb and index finger at mouth corners, making circles on the face as you visualize the sides of the face widening.

Go to the burn and make quick circles for a count of 20.

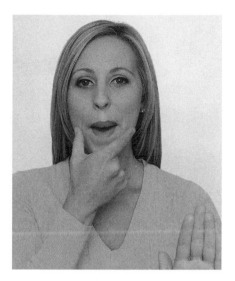

Exercise 5: The Cheek Energizer

Place one hand on wall or work surface, pushing away for resistance. Make a long, narrow oval shape with your mouth. Place thumb and index finger on cheeks. Smile with upper lip, keeping long oval shape and thinking the expression "Eww."

Repeat 10 times.

Move hand up middle of face, moving energy to top of head. Face forward, shoulders back. Push your feet against the floor for resistance. Pulse hand above head and hold for a count of 15.

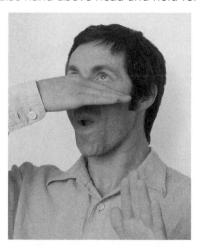
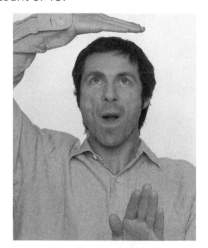

Exercise 6: The Nose Transformer

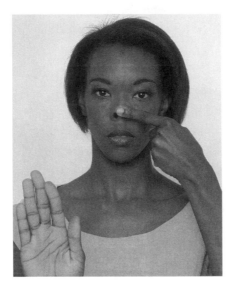

Place one hand on the wall or work surface, pushing away for resistance. Push your nose tip up hard with your index finger. Pull upper lip down and release.

Repeat 20 times.

Exercise 7: The Lip Lift

Place one hand on wall or work surface, pushing away for resistance. Close mouth. Tighten mouth corners. Visualize corners moving up and down. Use thumb and index fingers to track visualization of mouth corners. Push face forward, shoulders back. Hold until you feel a burn.

Pulse fingers and count to 30.

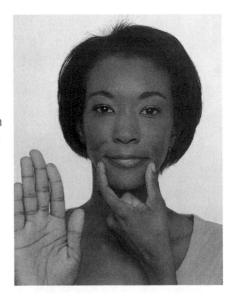

Exercise 8: The Lip Plumper

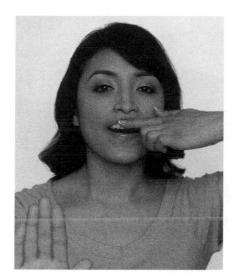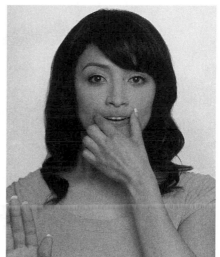

Place one hand on wall or work surface, pushing away for resistance. Curl your upper lip under. Push face forward, shoulders back. Visualize crushing a ball in center of lip. Tap center of lip with index finger. Make small circular movements until you feel a burn. Count to 20.

Tap corners of mouth with thumb and index finger. Make small circular movements until you feel a burn. Count to 20.

Exercise 9: The Nasolabial Plumper

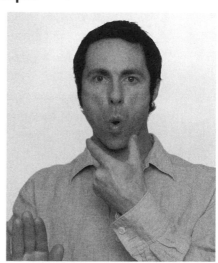

Place one hand on wall or work surface, pushing away for resistance. Make a long, narrow oval shape with your mouth. Push face forward, shoulders back. Place thumb and index fingers at mouth corners. Visualize energy moving up from mouth corners to nose corners. Visualize energy moving down from nose corners to mouth corners. Repeat until you feel a burn.

Pulse fingers for count of 30.

Exercise 10: The Neck Toner

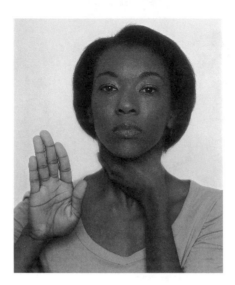

Place one hand on wall or work surface, pushing away for resistance. Place one hand on the front of your neck, as if you were choking yourself.

Push head away from body and release 20 times.

Exercise 11: The Jaw Toner

Place one hand on wall or work surface, pushing away for resistance. Roll your lower lip in over bottom teeth, wrap in mouth corners, pulling toward back teeth. Open and close jaw slowly five times. Tilt head up. Open and close jaw slowly five times, tilting head up. Hold. Push face forward, shoulders back. Starting at chin, move one hand up middle of face to top of head and pulse for count of 20.

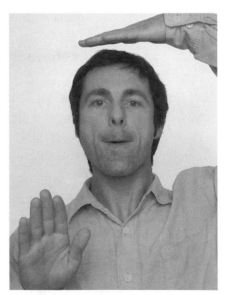

Exercise 12: The Face Contour

Place one hand on wall or work surface, pushing away for resistance. Open your mouth, roll your lips over the teeth and pull the mouth corners inside toward the back teeth. Visualize the sides of your face moving up along the sides of your head. Starting at the chin, use thumb and index finger of one hand and move up the sides of the face to top of the head as you visualize the sides lifting. Go until you feel the burn along the sides of face and pulse hand above head for count of 20.

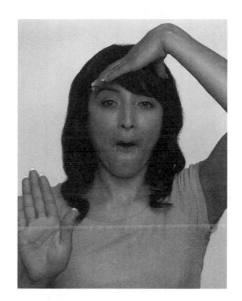

Exercise 13: The Neck and Chin Lift

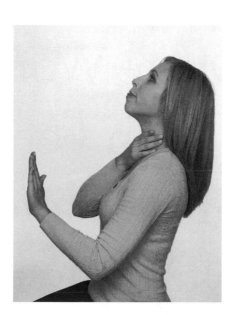

Place one hand on wall or work surface, pushing away for resistance. Place one hand on neck, chin up high. Smile with tongue pointing toward nose. Sit tall. Push away from wall like a rocking chair for 20 rocks. Turn head over right shoulder – 20 rocks. Turn head over left shoulder – 20 rocks.

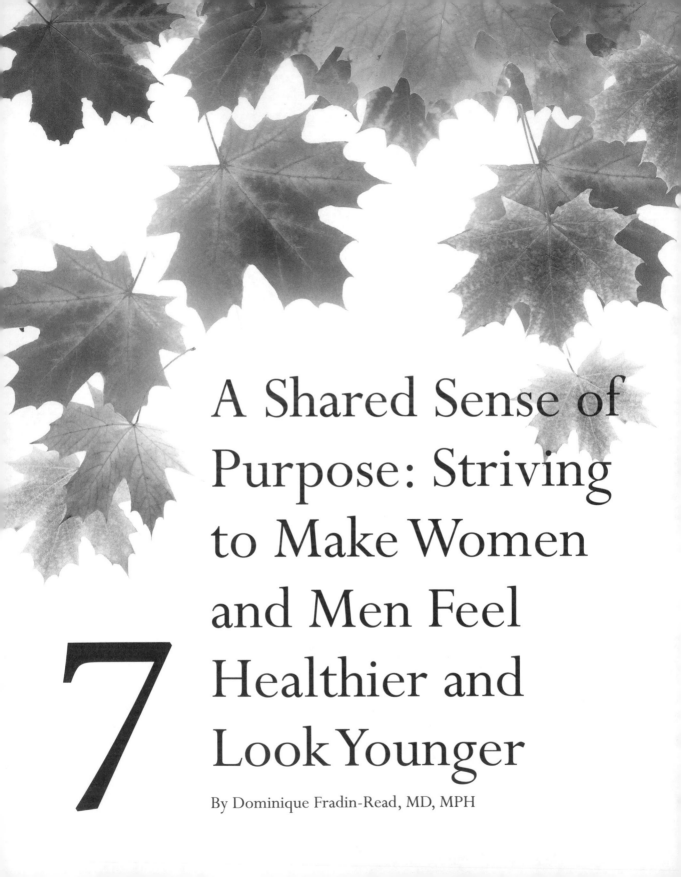

7

A Shared Sense of Purpose: Striving to Make Women and Men Feel Healthier and Look Younger

By Dominique Fradin-Read, MD, MPH

When I first met Carole Maggio, it was a true revelation! I had finally found a professional aesthetic-care specialist who showed a genuine interest in understanding beauty from the inside out. I was immediately impressed, not only by her thorough research of the complex anatomy of the facial muscles but also by her complete knowledge and understanding of the various processes involved in aging – and her science-based approach to skincare.

Those are qualities required to be a good aesthetic doctor, but obviously not always demonstrated among skincare specialists. What is an aesthetic doctor? It is someone who specializes in treating appearance issues, with invasive methods such as plastic surgery, or noninvasive methods such as Facercise.

As I learned more about Carole's Facercise program, I was amazed to discover how closely aligned our philosophies about health and beauty were. I soon found that we also shared a compassion and dedication to helping our patients and clients. Suffice it to say, we most definitely spoke the same language! Carole is a true healer; she is often able to "diagnose" some age-related health issues, and even suggests interventions that could help her clients feel healthier and look younger. At the same time, she has a great sense of humility and always defers the final decision to a healthcare professional when making her health recommendations.

My goal in writing this chapter will not be to repeat the topics that have already been developed in previous chapters. Rather, I will support Carole's approach to health and aesthetics – in particular Facercise – as an integral part of an optimal beauty lifestyle program. I will also discuss what actually constitutes an integrative approach to health, antiaging and beauty.

The Link Between Optimal Health and Optimal Beauty

As a doctor working in the field of wellness and prevention, I have worked with many patients to help them optimize their overall health and well-being – and teach them how to live longer, healthier and more productive lives. I soon discovered that for most of my dear patients, the notion of "optimal beauty" was also part of their quest for "optimal health." Even those who were focusing on their health issues began to concentrate more on their appearance, once they had experienced a much-improved level of wellness. At this point, patients noticed that not only were they feeling better – with increased stamina and energy – but their skin also looked better, or their hair was no longer falling out. These clients started questioning me about ways to improve their skin condition even more, and asked me to help them look younger and preserve their beauty. Obviously beauty was part of optimal health!

I have had the chance to meet with many renowned dermatologists and doctors who specialize in aesthetic medicine, in both Europe and the United States. Many of these specialists were intrigued by the effects that general preventive and antiaging advice could have when combined with their own interventions.

We started working in close collaboration. My role was to optimize the general health of our patients, while my colleagues were performing the aesthetics and dermatological (skin) treatments and procedures. The results were amazing: The texture of patients' skin looked healthier, more plumped and hydrated; the treatment benefits lasted longer; and fewer Botox injections were needed. Furthermore, most patients admitted experiencing better results – they felt they looked even younger than when they previously had the same cosmetic procedures or treatments performed *without* addressing their overall health.

Both patients and doctors admitted that restoring overall health from the inside out had indeed created better outcomes in terms of aesthetic appearance. Good health was undeniably an essential component to reaching optimal beauty.

Prevention and Regeneration

Several aesthetic-medicine academies currently exist in the United States and across the world. All of these organizations focus on local treatments and procedures, such as Botox toxin injections, fillers, laser therapy, chemical and mechanical resurfacing as well as cosmeceuticals (such as antiaging creams).

These types of treatments might have a temporary impact and give a younger-looking appearance for several months or years. None of them, however, offers an integrative approach that would:

- *Prevent* the process of aging
- *Restore* healthier body functions that support youth and beauty (for example, your metabolism or the way your hormones operate)
- *Address and harness* the regenerative abilities that adult skin cells and hair follicles possess in healthy conditions (in other words, skin and hair can regenerate when the body reaches optimal health)

The concept of prevention and regeneration started to make more sense to me as a growing number of patients began to look for more natural ways to stay healthy and preserve their youthful appearance. I had previous experience in Europe, working as the medical director of one of the major health spas in the South of France, where natural treatments – including a mineral-spring-water facial wash and algae applications – were used to restore overall skin health. I decided to study the various ways that we could use to slow down the aging process, as well as the methods and treatments that would support natural tissue rejuvenation. My findings were fascinating. Based on strong evidence and recent scientific data, I was able to design a preventive and regenerative model of care that could be offered as an alternative aesthetic-medicine approach – or combined with the current aesthetic treatments listed above to make them more effective. In particular, healthy lifestyle choices and exercise play an important role in the rejuvenation process – one reason why Facercise is an essential component of my program.

INTEGRATING PREVENTION AND REGENERATION

Goals

- Prevent
- Restore
- Regenerate

A Comprehensive Model of Care

- Encouraging a healthy lifestyle, including Facercise and anti-inflammatory detox
- Natural supplements, tailored to the individual for beauty, skin and hair support; general well-being; and change-of-lifestyle support
- Optimizing hormonal function
- Skincare products and facials
- New medical techniques to encourage optimal skin regeneration

Lifestyle Changes and Detoxing – The Ultimate Antiaging Agents

The role of lifestyle choices in overall health and aging has been clearly demonstrated. I could talk about the benefits of healthy lifestyle choices forever. I consider my role as not just that of a doctor, but also an educator. For this reason, it's important to pass on the latest medical knowledge and scientific discoveries in order to empower each of you, and help you understand how and why you can stay young and beautiful, and live longer, healthier lives.

I had the opportunity to enroll in the medical residency program in preventive medicine at Loma Linda University, California, where researchers are fully immersed in studying and teaching the effects of lifestyles on health. Loma Linda is one of the "Blue Zones" in the world, where people tend to live to be a healthy 100 years old at twice the rate of the rest of the world. It was interesting for me to discover that some population characteristics can predict health and longevity; these are natural healthy lifestyle practices that *everyone* can adopt. Genetic factors account for only about one-third of the problems associated with aging, while lifestyle factors contribute to two-thirds.

This leads me to the science of "epigenetics," an exciting field that has grown swiftly over the past several years. Epigenetics literally means "in addition to the genes," so it looks at the huge range of issues that can change the way our genes work, without actually changing the chromosomes we inherited from our parents. In other words, epigenetics focuses on the way the genes *behave*, not their structure. The DNA of your chromosomes remains the same, but your genes function *differently*. That's good news when it comes to aging.

A wide variety of illnesses and health issues have already been linked with epigenetic factors. These include almost all types of cancer; metabolic disorders; cardiovascular, autoimmune and emotional illnesses; and even cognitive function. The role of epigenetics in the aging process is an emerging field that promises exciting revelations in the near future; steadily increasing numbers of medical papers are now published in the area.

The consequences of epigenetic changes on skin aging are under particular scrutiny. One recent interesting study tried to identify the environmental factors that contribute to facial aging in identical twins. Smoking and sun exposure were strongly associated with an older appearance, dark, patchy skin discoloration and increased wrinkles. Twins who used hormone replacement therapy (HRT) had a younger appearance and more, better quality hair. This study offers strong evidence to show that it isn't just genes that affect the way our faces age; lifestyle plays a strong role. Additional studies are underway to further explain the processes involved in aging, and identify ways to reverse those processes.

What everyone needs to know is that *we are responsible for how our genes work*, and that *the way we treat our genes* can have a tremendous impact on our lives – and even our children's lives – and also affect the speed at which we age. There is a normal system in place inside our cells, which is designed to keep our "good genes" running and to suppress the "bad genes." Our lifestyle can have a huge influence on how the system works. Our food choices, exercise and sleep patterns, stress levels, exposure to toxins, environmental factors, hormonal status, and even our relationships and social interactions all have a dramatic effect on our gene function and overall health. All these factors also have a huge impact on our aging process and lifespan. Therefore, preserving the normal function of our genes is essential for preserving youth and beauty.

Nutrition

In particular, nutrition can subtly influence the reprogramming function of our genes. Recent studies suggest that some foods are able to turn on the "good genes," while others shut down these genes and activate the "bad" ones. You will not be surprised to hear that good epigenetic foods are fish, fruits and vegetables, nuts, omega-3 fatty acids (found in fish oils, for example), calcium-rich foods and whole grains. Bad epigenetic foods include red, processed and grilled meat, animal fat and hydrogenated fats (otherwise known as "trans fats"). Some components of food are also known to have protective effects – and might even change poor gene patterns to restore normal gene function. In particular, polyphenols and flavonoids, which are found in cruciferous vegetables (such as cabbage, turnips and broccoli), berries, grapes, citrus fruits and onions are good examples of healthy foods that can protect against cellular damage. Green tea, which we now know can suppress inflammation in the body, affects a protein found in our genes, which actually regulates the life cycle of a skin cell.

Grapes are rich in a natural chemical called resveratrol, which plays an important role in metabolic functions, supports cellular energy and weight loss, and has numerous beneficial actions to prevent cell death and prolong life.

Exercise

Researchers in the UK recently studied the facial images of women who looked young and confirmed that a youthful appearance was linked to the structure of subcutaneous tissues – in a nutshell, the fitness and tone of the facial muscles.

New discoveries now confirm that exercise reverses aging at the gene level. The genes involved are responsible for the function of the mitochondria, which are in charge of the energy and growth of the cells. Mitochondria have been described as the "powerhouse" of the cells; they play a major role in protecting the cells against aging. Problems with the mitochondria can lead to the loss of muscle mass and strength as we age.

A recent experiment analyzed tissue samples of muscle cells of healthy older men and women before and after a regular six-month exercise program, and compared the results to those of younger adults. The results confirmed that mitochondrial function declines with age. *However,* after exercise there was a remarkable reversal of the process, and the mitochondrial function returned to levels similar to those of younger adults. This confirms that exercise clearly protects against the age-related decline of both muscle mass and muscle strength by acting at the core level of the genes. Therefore, it is logical to conclude that the Facercise program can help our mitrochondrial function return to levels similar to those of younger adults. Sounds complicated? It is not, really. Basically, exercising the facial muscles will have an antiaging impact on your face as a whole.

Toxins

Factors that negatively affect the skin – and promote the aging process – include heavy metals, pesticides, diesel exhaust, tobacco smoke, alcohol, radioactivity, viruses and bacteria. Of course, the best way to stay healthy is to avoid exposure to these toxins, quit smoking and limit alcohol intake.

Unfortunately, there is no doubt that our modern world is becoming increasingly toxic and it is almost impossible to be totally protected. These toxins can accumulate as they move up the food chain, and it seems that a cocktail of toxins is much more powerful than its individual parts; in other words, together, the toxins we breathe, absorb and eat are much more powerful as a group.

Many of these substances induce a chronic inflammatory response in the body that can have harmful consequences, such as cancer, cardiovascular, reproductive, metabolic, dermatological and mental health disorders to name just a few, and can accelerate the damaging effects of aging.

As a result, many alternative practitioners recommend something called a "xenobiotic detoxification" (basically a program to rid your body of poisons); however, I need to warn you against the huge number of products that claim to have detox properties but are not proven to be effective and can be potentially harmful. Any anti-inflammatory detoxification program should be performed under the supervision of a trained healthcare professional.

A good product needs to be scientifically designed to address the various phases of the detoxification process. Turmeric, alpha-lipoic acid (ALA), glutathione and N-acetylcysteine are phytochemicals (plant chemicals) that have been proven to work at cell level and can safely and effectively be included in a detox. Plants such as milk thistle, artichoke and berberine are also proven to be helpful by supporting the liver during the detoxification process.

Most of my patients understand the need to add a safe detoxification program to their health-maintenance regimen, particularly when their goal is to prevent disease and experience antiaging benefits. Immediate results can usually be seen on your skin, which becomes clearer and smoother. Most patients with acne will see a drastic reduction in the number of spots and lesions on their face.

For a comprehensive approach to a detoxification program, lymphatic drainage and saunas can be added and used to effectively mobilize fat-soluble toxins or poisons.

Other Factors

I would like to emphasize the essential role played by restorative sleep and the importance of respecting normal biological rhythms. These have been found to have a strong impact on the health of our genes, and to help reverse the degenerative effects of aging.

In addition, skin nutraceuticals (nutritional products that offer health and medical benefits to the skin), as well as vitamins and natural supplements to prevent aging, have shown substantial benefits when used wisely and appropriately. A good physician can help you identify them. In general, however, a whole, balanced and varied diet should provide most of the nutrients.

If you do wish to add supplements to ensure that your body gets what it needs to function at an optimal level – and help change the way your genes operate – it is important to see a qualified practitioner. It really is vital that you get the correct dose of any supplement *for you*. For example, vitamin D, when taken at the right dosage, is known to delay the aging process, protect against skin cancer and encourage the growth cycle of your hair follicles. However, if taken in excess, it can cause premature aging. Unfortunately, there is no one-dose-fits-all recommendation for this vitamin. You'll need to have a blood test done and the adequate dose prescribed for you, according to your needs.

I am always concerned when patients arrive in my office with bags or bottles of supplements, purchased on the basis of potentially unsound advice. They often do not realize that the recommended products contain overlapping formulas of similar ingredients, and that the final daily intake of certain vitamins or essential nutrients far exceeds the maximum health safety threshold. In addition, many people are unaware of the risks of the non-active ingredients added to these products. My position is clear: only hypoallergenic pharmaceutical-grade supplements should be used, with no added coatings, binders, shellacs, artificial flavors, artificial sweeteners, colorings or fragrances that would disrupt the action of any of the active ingredients.

HELPING YOU STAY MOTIVATED

When appropriately prescribed, specific mood-enhancing natural supplements can also be extremely helpful for supporting your motivation during the process of changing your lifestyle. Most people have a fairly clear idea of what good nutrition is – as well as how much we should exercise. So why is it so hard to implement healthy lifestyle changes?

If you've struggled unsuccessfully to improve your lifestyle, you'll be happy to know that I do not believe in willpower alone. I believe that the mind and the chemistry of your body need to be balanced before changes can begin, and be successfully maintained.

By choosing the right "cocktail" of safe, natural, anti-stress supplements, also called adaptogens, which are able to optimize your inner strength and energy, you'll find it dramatically easier to change your behavior, make the right food choices and start enjoying the practice of regular exercise.

Is Optimizing Your Hormones the Key to the Fountain of Youth?

Hormones are powerful chemical substances produced by specific glands and cells in the body, and carried by the bloodstream to the target cells. Hormones are essential to life; some decline with age, others might increase abnormally. In healthy young people, hormones work in harmony in the body, where they regulate various physiological activities. Estrogen, progesterone, testosterone, thyroid hormones, growth hormone, cortisol and insulin are all involved in some way in the aging process. What's more, melatonin has recently been identified as having a potential role in the way our genes operate.

As we age, hormonal imbalances can occur, and these imbalances may be the reason why some of us do not feel well and why our energy levels decline. Such imbalances are implicated in numerous symptoms and diseases that occur with age, including heart disease, cancer, metabolic disorders and weight gain, immune dysfunction, osteoporosis, cognitive impairment and depression. The skin is one of the largest organs of the body and is significantly affected by hormonal changes. Fluctuations in hormone levels at certain periods of life, such as menopause, can have a tremendous impact on the skin, hair and nails.

If you would like to evaluate your hormones, I strongly recommend that you work with a trained preventive health/antiaging doctor, as an effective antiaging program requires that all of your hormones be adjusted to a safe and optimal level. Synthetic products for menopause, including HRT, have acquired bad press after the publication of the Women's Health Initiative study, which pointed out their risks – particularly when taken orally and prescribed for patients with identified health risks (women who smoke, are overweight, or suffer from high blood pressure). Since then, the use of bioidentical hormones (natural substances that are chemically identical to hormones) has been found to be a good alternative. Each woman is unique with her own risk profile and preferences; therefore, individual treatment is the key to provide maximum health benefits and minimum health risks.

In my practice I have been prescribing hormonal treatments to a number of peri- and post-menopausal women – as well as to men undergoing andropause changes (the equivalent of a male menopause). All of them reported improvement in their overall health. The benefits are numerous, such as improved general energy levels, restoration of normal sleep, decrease in sugar cravings and regulation of food intake, increased motivation to exercise, decreased bloating, weight loss, positive mood changes, and obvious signs of skin and hair rejuvenation.

What About the Future?

The new science of epigenetics is leading researchers to discover innovative antiaging methods and technologies, and to propose specific treatments and therapies that can slow down or reverse the negative effects of age-related gene changes. This will help each of us look and stay young for longer. Alongside this, other investigators are focusing on the use of stem cells and extracts of stem-cell mediums for skin and hair rejuvenation. Some products are already available in Europe and Asia; others are currently being investigated in clinical trials. Preliminary results are extremely encouraging and such treatments should be available soon.

Cell Therapy: Promises for the Future

By Judy Smith, wife of the late Dr. C. Tom Smith

My husband, the late Dr. C. Tom Smith, was Medical Director of the International Clinic for Biological Regeneration (ICBR) from 1981 until his recent passing. ICBR practices cell therapy at clinics in London, the Bahamas and Mexico. Although cell therapy is utilized in Europe and many other nations, it is not yet FDA-approved for use in the United States. But one form of cell therapy practiced every day in the United States is blood transfusion – as well as red and white blood cell therapy. On a less frequent basis, bone marrow transplant or thymus cell implant are also practiced.

Live cell therapy was developed in the early 1930s by Dr. Paul Niehans (1882–1971), a Swiss doctor who became known as the "father of cell therapy." Cell therapy using sheep cells can do many wonderful things for the body. It can strengthen the immune system, increase energy levels and keep the cells more youthful.

Dr. Smith became interested in live cell therapy after he was involved in a very serious radiation accident, where his thyroid was exposed to high levels of radiation. After the accident he was given a six-month life expectancy. Due to the damage to his thyroid, he experienced various health problems, including cancer and increased biological aging. As a result, he became interested in various antiaging options. Ultimately, he modeled his therapies on Dr. Paul Niehans' method of live cell therapy, which he administered at his La Prairie Clinic in Switzerland.

Dr. Niehans once stated the goal of cell therapy in this way: "What I am striving after is not only to give more years to life but especially to give more life to years." In keeping with this, cell therapists have reported that their patients' skin tone and complexion improves, their vitality increases, their youthful optimism and energy returns, and various other conditions of aging much improve. The future holds unlimited promise for cell therapy.

WHAT IS CELL THERAPY?

Cell therapy is the injection of cells or tissues from animal organs (sheep) in a physiological solution. Its benefits are many but, essentially, doctors who practice cell therapy believe it acts like an organ transplant and makes the old cells "act younger." It is used for the treatment of loss of vitality; physical and mental exhaustion; convalescence after illness; premature aging; signs of deterioration of the brain, heart, kidneys, lungs, liver and digestive organs; lack of drive and declining mental efficiency; weak immune system; arthritis and other degenerative diseases; endocrine dysfunction and menopausal disturbances; Parkinson's; and chronic pain, brain, heart and circulatory issues. Fundamentally, cell therapy has been shown to successfully revitalize and extend youthfulness.

Client Testimonials

Dearest Carole,

Words are inadequate to express the gratitude I feel for you because of the transformation that has occurred in my life since I began your fabulous Facercise program. During my forties and early fifties I felt very stressed and overwhelmed. About three years ago, I hit rock bottom when I thought I was having a heart attack! One of my sons, Nathan, drove me to the emergency room where I continued getting sick to my stomach for over 12 hours. This was truly an aha moment for me. I decided then and there that life is too short and precious to waste. I needed to begin life anew, take charge of my life, explore new options and make some positive changes.

Besides taking better care of myself, reducing my stress, eating better and working out, I wanted to do something about my face. Research has always been my asset, so I checked out yours and other facial exercise programs. Facercise appeared to be the most effective and definitely the most impressive one on several levels. One, you personally demonstrated it, and that proves it works; two, it has longevity – it has been around for over 20 years; and three, it was the only one in which you experience lactic-acid burn in the facial muscles.

Last year, at age 56, I impulsively decided to enter the *More* magazine / Wilhelmina Model Search for Women Over 40 contest. I had no expectations, but decided to take the chance anyway. My daughter said to me, "Oh, Mom, there will be thousands of beautiful women entering." I didn't even bother to tell my sons. I dropped off a picture that had been taken a year earlier (pre-Facercise) by a professional photographer. I guess I was above-average looking when I was chosen as one of the 10 finalists out of over 16,000 women. However, when I arrived in New York

I think they were very surprised to see the new me! By this time I had been faithfully using your Facercise program and had blossomed intensely! My skin was toned and radiant. Everyone commented on how beautiful I was, how beautiful my skin and neck were, etc. And do you know, I was the oldest of all the finalists! In fact, 15 years older than most! I remember one of the journalists from *More* magazine asked me if I would ever consider having "anything done" — that is, plastic surgery. I told her that I would never need to have anything done because I'd found Facercise!

The Facercise program has truly transformed my life. I never felt or thought of myself as beautiful until I began using your program. I love being in my fifties and look forward to each new decade now that I have found the secret to a youthful face. I feel intensely youthful in spirit, appearance and enthusiasm. I'm on an exciting journey, and for the first time, I feel that I have unlimited opportunities and potential to do and be anything I choose.

Thank you again for your life's work and support of women. You will always be at the top of my gratitude list.

All my best,
Pamela Kelley Leitzell
Houston, Texas

Hello Carole,

I want to start off by saying that when I first discovered Facercise I was very skeptical that it would be able to help me. I thought that the "before" and "after" pictures on the website were misleading because the lighting seemed different, or that they were tilting their heads in such a way to make it appear that they were getting results. I then thought that perhaps they had had cosmetic procedures done. *Boy, was I ever wrong!*

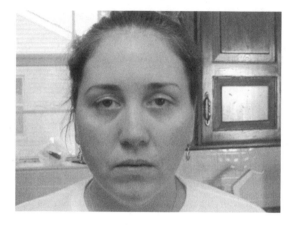 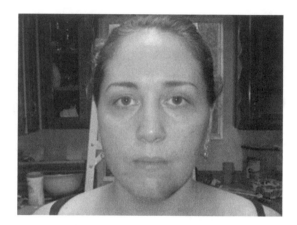

Just to give you a little background about myself: I went through a very painful breakup with a man I had been with for almost eight years. I really started to age very rapidly from the stress and depression, and in a very short time my face began to drop. I also gained a considerable amount of weight during this time. I have been starting to feel better and have recently gone on a diet and decided that if I was to be working out my body, I needed to include my face as well. I have been doing the Facercise program for about two to three weeks now. I only performed the exercises the way I was supposed to for about three days but then got lazy and just did them here and there. I didn't really think anything was happening and was about to give up when I decided to go ahead and take some more pictures to see if I could notice even a tiny improvement. I was not expecting to see what I saw! As you can see in the pictures, my eyes are definitely opening up and the hollows and darkness beneath my eyes has improved. I had some puffiness under my bottom lip and that has gone down dramatically! My mouth corners are turning up, my naso-labial creases are gone and I can see that my face is starting to lift. I am so excited about what I am seeing! I am almost 37 and I am hoping that within the next six months, my face will look even better than when I was 25! Thank you so much for this wonderful gift! I want others to know how fabulous this program really is! Even though I do not have the full results just yet, I am feeling and seeing an undeniable difference and it makes me so very happy!

Many blessings,
Tracy from Texas :)

• •

Dear Carole,

I have been using the new Ultimate Facercise DVD for a little over a month now. I wanted to write and tell you how happy I am with my results so far. I believe my overall look has "softened" a bit. My eyes are a bit larger, and my right eyebrow has lifted – it was definitely droopy prior to Facercise! My neck has improved as well as the area just below my neck, as my collarbones are not as visible. Also, the furrows between my brows have nearly disappeared! I will continue to work the program because I know I can and will achieve the results I want. I just need to work a little longer. Thanks for developing a program that can truly reverse the signs of aging naturally!

Many thanks
Debbie Todd
Cape Coral, Florida

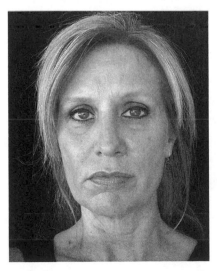

Debbie, pre-Facercise

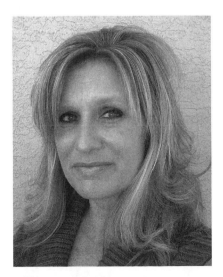

Debbie, post-Facercise

Dear Carole,

I turned 45 in March 2009 and, yes, I was starting to show the signs of aging. In the first photo, you can see that there was a lot of wagging, sagging and dragging going on. I was starting to look like a deflated blowfish and I absolutely hated my profile. I had actually begun flirting with the idea of getting a Lifestyle Lift when, just by chance, I found your Facercise book. I read the book and thought to myself, "What the heck, I'll give it a try." After all, I had nothing to lose and everything to gain – "if it actually works," that is!

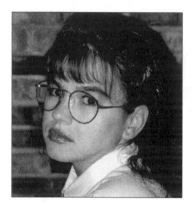

Sharon, age 30

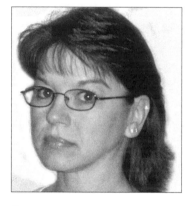

Sharon, age 46

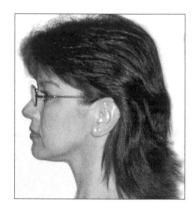

Sharon, age 46

So I took this "before" picture to be able to monitor any changes in my appearance. It is said that a picture is worth a thousand words, and ain't that the truth! In the "before" picture, you can see that my jawline was a droopy mess, and what was under my chin was in fact another chin. I called it my "dangling participle." Now, take a good look at the "after" photo. You can clearly see that my extra chin has almost completely disappeared. My jawline is smoothing out and my cheeks are back where they belong. My face is being restored to a much healthier look and feel. I no longer have that tired, frumpy, droopy look going on! My face is actually changing and looking more and more like it used to before gravity slapped me in the face – literally! I'm also including a picture taken when I was 30 and today at age 46 (front and side views) to demonstrate how Facercise is keeping me youthful-looking.

When I started out, I was doing all of the exercises excluding the Face Widener [The Face Filler; see page 65]. I was about two and a half weeks into the program when I noticed that my lips were becoming a little too plump, so I backed off from practicing that [Lip Plumper] exercise. I love the fact that I can pick and choose which improvements and changes I want to make to my face. Surgery would not have allowed that, plus it would have cost me up the yin-yang – not to mention the pain! I am really looking forward to watching how my face will improve as time marches on. It had been marching right across my face for quite a while!

*See Sharon's "before" photos on page 16, including one that she considers to be "a work in progress."

The reason I took the time to write to you is because of all the naysayers. Many people will slam your program without ever trying it, and that just doesn't seem right. By using Facercise, I am restructuring my face, but I am doing it the natural way. It doesn't hurt a bit and there is no costly investment, no downtime and that is a huge plus! Thank you, Carole, for sharing your program!*

Sincerely,
Sharon Martin
Murray, Utah

• •

Hi Carole,

I am 44 years old and all of the females in my family are prone to jowls and loose skin on our necks. I also have excessive under-eye puffiness. I have been doing your new Ultimate Facercise program for just 15 days now and all I can say is *WOW*!!! My jowls and neck are firming up and the puffiness under my eyes is going away. Facercise is going to override heredity. I am amazed. Thank you so much, Carole!

Sincerely,
Linda James
Chicago, Illinois

• •

Dear Carole,

The idea of working out my face muscles made sense to me. After all, I went to the gym to work out arms and legs, why not the face? I had a problem, not a major one, just something that kind of annoyed me. My eyes drooped. Actually, drooping eyes didn't bother me, what was really annoying was how many people during the course of the day would ask me, "Are you tired?" Not only did my eyes droop, but my right eyelid was a bit lazy. In fact, I had this lazy eyelid for as far back as I can remember, and every now and then – perhaps when I really got tired – the eyelid would remind me it was lazy by developing a slight tic. It was nothing serious, just a little twitch to make my day more tedious.

By luck, I came across your *Facercise* book. I admit I was a bit skeptical at first. I read the book, stared at the images, but still wasn't sure I was doing the exercises right. Not to mention that I felt kind of silly trying to "feel the burn" in my cheeks. Still, the idea made sense, so I gave it a chance. After a week or so, something happened. People started to ask me what I had done. "Were you tanning?" asked one. "You lost weight," insisted another. I barely noticed, but within a short while, people were noticing something different and it was definitely positive.

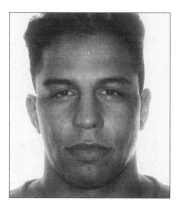   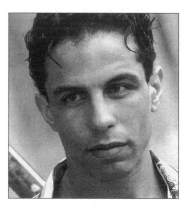

Matt, pre-Facercise   Matt, post-Facercise

By toning, shaping and strengthening the dozens of muscles that form the human face, Facercise was slowly and naturally changing my facial features – for the better. My eyes were wider, more open and alert. My jawline was sharper, my lips firmed up and even my hairline seemed to come down. Best of all, I actually liked doing the exercises. A two-minute workout in the shower in the morning helped to shake off that morning grogginess. A quick midday session actually relieved stress (who knew the face could carry stress?).

I've always been a kind of self-help guy, and that's exactly what your program offered me. Facercise is a way of allowing me to improve myself by letting my face reflect how I really feel – happy.

Sincere thanks,
Matt Sanchez
Los Angeles, California

Dear Ms. Maggio,

I purchased your books (both Facercise and Facebuilder) about two months ago, and have been working out my face on a daily basis ever since. I feel I have rejuvenated my face by at least 10 years! I am enclosing a photo that was taken five years ago — and a photo of how I look today.

My own mother said she cannot believe I am the same person! Please note that I am 36 and people used to guess my correct age. But today, when I ask someone I have just met to guess my age, they often guess 27, 28, 29. They cannot believe it when I tell them that I am actually almost ten years older.

Your program gave me that extra boost of confidence I was truly lacking. Today, I feel very much alive, confident, happier and stronger than ever before. Thank you very much for your wonderful programs, and please continue with your great work.

Best regards,
Noël Maasdam
The Netherlands

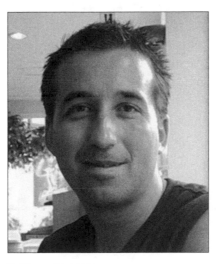

Noël, pre-Facercise

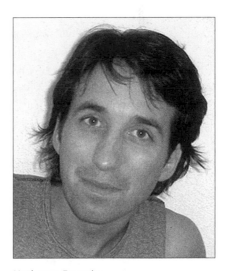

Noël, post-Facercise

Professional Testimonials

As a doctor certified in both preventive and antiaging medicine, I strongly believe in the benefits of Facercise to slow down the aging process. Every day in my practice I meet patients who are looking for natural ways to help them stay healthy and preserve their youthful appearance. They express their concern and disappointment regarding the limited options offered by most cosmetic medicine physicians – repeated Botox toxin injections, fillers and/or plastic-surgery procedures – as the only viable treatment choices available. Motivated to change the current model toward healthy aging, prevention and rejuvenation, I started working in close collaboration with Carole Maggio. Both of us share the same goal: to slow down the aging process naturally and help restore the regenerative capacity of a healthy, young-looking face and body. Facercise is not just an exercise program for the facial muscles; it is an essential part of a comprehensive approach to health and beauty that also includes protective lifestyle recommendations, appropriate antiaging nutrient support and optimal, individualized hormonal balance. Many of my patients have already experienced the benefits of the program, enjoying a smoother, plumper skin texture, a lifting effect of the muscles of the face, decreased sagging cheeks and an overall younger shape of the face.

Recent scientific data now supports the evidence that exercise addresses the aging processes directly at the chromosome level of the muscle cells. Tissue samples taken from muscle after exercise demonstrate a remarkable reversal of the genetic fingerprint back to levels similar to those seen in younger adults. To me, there is no doubt that a comprehensive rejuvenation approach for the face should incorporate a well-structured exercise program. Facercise is the answer. Every exercise described in the book has been thoroughly studied, and every technique is designed to help the client reach their maximum potential facial fitness goals. I am personally using the

Facercise program every day, and I am grateful that Carole Maggio has taken me on this fascinating and rejuvenating journey

Sincerely,
Dominique Fradin-Read, MD, MPH
Santa Monica, California

Interview with Dr. Vince Marcel, chiropractor and nutritional counselor, El Segundo, California, by journalist Averie Benet

AB: Hello, Doctor, and thank you for your time today to speak with me about Carole Maggio. When did you first meet Carole?

Dr. Marcel: Well, I first met Carole a number of years ago at a women's healthcare fundraiser we held at my clinic in El Segundo, where Carole gave a very inspirational presentation. I'm a chiropractor and we treat patients not only with chiropractic adjustments, but also nutritional-response testing and counseling, acupuncture, detoxification programs as well as hyperbaric chamber treatments.

AB: So obviously you are very aware of the effect that nutrition, as well as stress, plays in the overall health of the body.

Dr. Marcel: I am. Nutrition is so important to your overall health and well-being, as well as the proper nutrition for your blood type.

AB: When was the next time you saw her?

Dr. Marcel: The next time we reconnected was after I found out I had Bell's palsy.

AB: Would you mind sharing the details of your story with me?

Dr. Marcel: About five months ago, we were having an office party. I was eating my lunch when all of the sudden I felt like an 80-year-old person, chewing my food with dentures. I just couldn't seem to chew properly. My tongue began to tingle, as though I'd just had a Novocain shot. Then my right eye began to tear uncontrollably, as though I had been exposed to some really strong perfume. Obviously I knew something was terribly wrong and started to think that perhaps I was having a stroke. I knew I needed a good cervical adjustment, but I couldn't give one to myself.

So, I went see a medical doctor who happens to be a friend of mine.

There is no specific laboratory test to confirm diagnosis of the disorder. She went through a number of physical evaluations to test for upper and lower facial weakness and to rule out other possibilities. She told me that I did not have Bell's palsy.

Later that evening, my right eye became even more irritated and began to swell up. Suddenly, I noticed that I couldn't raise my right eyebrow. By this time, it was getting late and I was rather exhausted. Only now I could not close my right eye. It was around 1:30 a.m. when I decided to tape my eye closed in order to get some sleep.

Within the next few days I went to see three different specialists. I saw a homeopathic chiropractor, who had just finished working with his assistant who had Bell's palsy. He was convinced I had Bell's. He did some tests and determined I had some toxicity in my body. I was not that surprised, as six weeks prior I had suffered from food poisoning, so I concluded this could be related. I knew my body was in a weakened state from the food toxin and felt my nervous system had also been overtaxed. I went to see an acupuncturist who also had experience with Bell's palsy patients. By now, I had lost all function on the right side of my face. I could *feel* the right side of my face, but had absolutely no control over the muscles at all. I could no longer close my lips. If I closed my left eye, my right eye remained open. If I smiled, the left side of my mouth would turn up; on the right side nothing would happen. The right side was completely deadened. My face was flaccid and when I looked in the mirror, I saw the face of a stroke patient.

My wife and I returned to the medical doctor when I was at my worst. She then agreed that I indeed had Bell's palsy and prescribed several medications – one to reduce swelling and one to combat the side effect of a potential stomach ulcer from the first medication. I declined to take the medications since my stomach was already in bad shape from the food poisoning. Instead I decided to take homeopathic medicine, which would address the issues without all of the side effects.

Next I saw a nutritionist, who sent me home with many different supplements and vitamins to try to get my body back to normal. For the first time, I started seeing some changes. After five days had passed, I had a phone consultation with another medical doctor, who recommended a steroid injection. However, I declined since I knew that the window had already closed. You see, normally a steroid injection should be administered within 72 hours of the onset of symptoms in order for it to be effective. I decided to return to my homeopath, who used laser therapy on me, and I went for some more acupuncture treatments. But nothing I did would restore my face. I still had virtually no control over the muscles on the right side of my face. It was then that I decided to call Carole.

AB: Why Carole? And why did you think she could help you?

Dr. Marcel: I knew that she had a unique perspective and intense knowledge of the anatomy of the face. I also knew I needed an expert in facial therapy and rehabilitation to help me get my face back to feeling and looking normal again. So I called her and we arranged to meet at her spa on her day off.

AB: What happened during your meeting or session?

Dr. Marcel: Well, she worked with me intensely for an hour. It was really very taxing on me and, by the end of our session, I was completely exhausted.

AB: Did she create a special program just for you?

Dr. Marcel: Absolutely.

AB: Can you tell me about your results?

Dr. Marcel: My wife and I went to see Carole at least four or five times in the beginning, and then I would do the exercises every morning and evening. I have to say that the results were truly amazing. They were amazing to me because, remember, I had virtually no muscle control. None. Zero on the right side of my face. It felt as if my face was completely frozen on the right side. I almost felt like I'd been given an overdose of a Botox injection. It was weird because I could "feel" the right side of my face, but had absolutely no control over the muscles. But then something miraculous happened. By day three, I started to feel a twitching sensation above my right nostril. This was definitely a sign of hope for me. After I did the exercises one evening, my wife noticed an immediate improvement. She said she could see lines appear on my forehead. While this may not seem positive to some, it is for a

Bell's palsy patient whose face was previously frozen. By day four, I was able to close my right eye. I would say that by the one-week mark, I was about 75 percent improved. It was truly amazing to me. I was able to squint again and raise my eyebrow up.

After three weeks' time, I had 90 percent full facial functionality back. I could speak better, had more energy, and didn't get quite as exhausted by the end of the day. By the six-week mark, I was 95 percent of the way back to normal. By Christmas day, I was able to smile and both sides of my mouth went up. This was a wonderful improvement for me and my wife and kids to see.

AB: Do you still do the exercises today, Dr. Marcel?

Dr. Marcel: Oh, absolutely. They've helped me so much in my journey back to normalcy and, really, it only takes me about six minutes a day to do them. That's the beautiful thing about the program. I notice that I can actually see the corners of my eye crinkle again and that's a good thing because that means I can squint. The exercise program Carole created for me was my saving grace. I am ever so grateful to Carole; she is a kind and caring person who really has an in-depth knowledge about the facial muscles – but, more importantly, she has a deep passion to help people. I thank God every day that she is in my life.

About the Author

Carole Maggio is a licensed aesthetician, spa owner and bestselling author, whose books are sold worldwide. Facercise was developed by Carole Maggio more than 30 years ago and is widely accepted as an excellent alternative to cosmetic surgery. Facercise has twice been named as one of the top 100 beauty products in the world, and Carole Maggio has been called the world's foremost authority on facial exercises.

Facercise has been used for years by rock stars, royalty, politicians, celebrities, business leaders, sports figures, doctors and dentists.

For information about DVDs, web-cam classes, seminars or Carole's world-renowned skincare line, call 1-800-597-3555 (or 1-310-316-1818 in California). Fax number: 1-310-540-8048.

You can also visit the Facercise website at www.facercise.com, or email Carole at cmaggio@facercise.com.

Carole's postal address is:
Carole Maggio Day Spa
1713 South Catalina Avenue
Redondo Beach, CA 90277

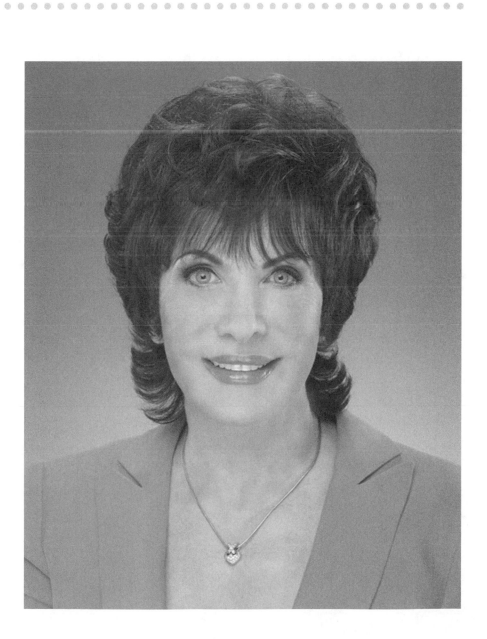

Dedication

I would like to dedicate this book to the legions of clients who have joined me in the fight to reverse the appearance and effects of the aging process. We are successfully changing the face and the pace of aging. My quest began quietly in 1981 and has advanced to a wave of worldwide recognition. With Facercise, we have shown that we can successfully turn back the hands of time.

I would like to express my love and eternal gratitude to my dear friend April, for all the support she has given me over many years. I would like to thank my husband, who has supported my efforts through thick and thin and who has always been there to cheer me on – and up, when the going gets tough.

I would also like to thank my wonderful staff at my spa. They keep things moving and grooving, even when I am not there.